FIVE MINUTES OF AMAZING

My journey through Dementia

At the age of thirty-eight, Chris Graham was diagnosed with a rare form of Alzheimer's disease that had already killed his father in his forties and put his brother in a nursing home aged forty-three. A long-serving British soldier, he'd recently discovered that his girlfriend Vicky was pregnant. He was faced with dismissal from the army on medical grounds and the terrible decision of whether to keep their unborn child, who had a 50 per cent chance of inheriting the dementia gene. After their son's birth, Chris embarked on a 10,000-mile solo cycle around North America raising money and awareness for Alzheimer's research.

FIVE MINUTES OF AMAZING

Five Minutes Of Amazing

My Race Against Dementia

by

Chris Graham with Wendy Holden

Magna Large Print Books
Long Preston, North Yorkshire,
BD23 4ND, England.

British Library Cataloguing in Publication Data.

A catalogue record of this book is
available from the British Library

ISBN   978-0-7505-4554-9

First published in Great Britain in 2016 by Sphere

Published in Large Print 2018 by arrangement with
Little, Brown Book Group Limited

Magna Large Print is an imprint of Library Magna Books Ltd.

Printed and bound in Great Britain by
T.J. (International) Ltd., Cornwall, PL28 8RW

'Chris is a great example of someone who, when faced with a difficult diagnosis, has shown extraordinary grit and determination to overcome his circumstances and ensure that future generations can benefit from potentially life-saving research.'

David Cameron

Contents

To my children Natalie, Marcus and Dexter, and to all those who are living with dementia and its consequences.

This memoir is based on my
recollection of events which may
not be as others recall them.

Where conversations cannot be
remembered precisely, I have re-created
them to the best of my ability.

Any mistakes are my own.

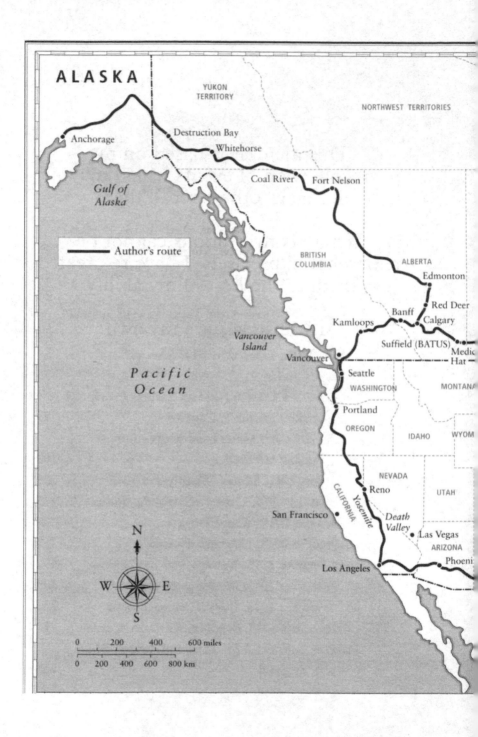

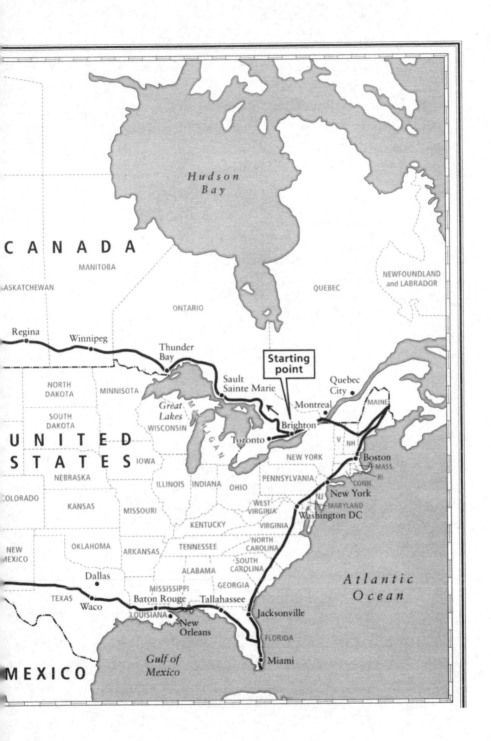

Prologue

'Success is not final. Failure is not fatal. It's the courage to continue that counts.'
WINSTON CHURCHILL

Dementia Adventure Diary, 4 May 2015, near Espanola, Ontario, Canada

It was past ten o'clock at night and I hadn't a Scooby-Doo where I was. After a tough twelve-hour day in the saddle, cycling more than 130 miles through rain, wind and sleet, I was tired, soaked through and miserable. A strong head-wind had been against me all day and my bum was in bits. My throat was parched and I longed to stop somewhere and prime the kettle for a cup of tea – my only vice.

My problem was that I'd cocked up big time. The campsite Vicky had suggested I aim for that night was twenty-five miles behind me after I'd decided that I could push myself further that day and wing it. 'I want to keep going,' I told her when she rang to find out why I was still on the road so late at night. 'My legs feel all right and I've had something to eat. There's bound to be another campsite somewhere up ahead, right?'

Wrong, soldier.

As it turned out there was nowhere else for several hundred miles, a fact of my ride that would become a frequent ordeal. I would have no choice but to wild camp by the side of the road in the dark despite the risk of bears, wolves and snakes.

I'd thought this cycling lark would be easy. Sitting on my arse all day – I mean, how hard could it be? But in taking on this endurance challenge I'd dubbed 'My Dementia Adventure: The Long Cycle Round', I'd swapped twenty-three years of soldiering for foul weather, winds whipping my face, and cruelly deceptive hills. Armed with a sturdy bike, a sense of humour, and some good old-fashioned British grit, I'd spent my days dodging dangerous wildlife and avoiding near misses with the giant metal monsters that ruled the roads.

Whenever the sun came out I'd be sweating like a moose on heat. Then sudden rains would drench me – something I thought I'd be used to coming from Manchester – but cycling when you're wet leads to some pretty unpleasant chafing, I can tell you. Not to mention saddle soreness.

Come back, Army life. All is forgiven.

'I should have planned better,' I complained to 'Shirley', my American-manufactured Surly bike, and the only one still listening. 'I should have done what Vicks said and checked ahead. She warned me not to try to go it alone. Better still, I should never have bloody decided to cycle around the whole of North America on my own in the first place!'

I thought of Vicky, nearly four thousand miles away back home near RAF Brize Norton in Oxfordshire. I knew she'd be worrying where on earth I was heading now as she followed my

18

signals on the satellite tracker. In between working as a part-time gardener, care worker, and studying for a photography diploma, she had our newborn baby Dexter and her eleven-year-old daughter Katy to care for. Our house was full of packing boxes from our recent move and she often had to stay up until three or four in the morning to be my unofficial 'Mission Control' at base camp. God love her.

From the moment I set eyes on Vicks, I knew we were meant to be together. After a fractured childhood, four years in a children's home and two broken marriages, at thirty-eight years old I needed some stability in my life. I just hadn't factored in all the other stuff that happened so soon after we met. Neither had Vicky. Incredibly, when she learned she was accidentally pregnant with Dexter and twenty-four hours later we were informed of the true severity of the sentence hanging over me, she barely flinched.

'I've probably only got a few good years left,' I reminded her, still reeling from the diagnosis. 'The doctors think I could be dead in seven.'

'So?' she said stoically. 'I'd rather have five minutes of amazing than a lifetime of never having met you.' And with that one declaration she refused to give up on me – or our unborn child.

Then, when I told her that I wanted to go ahead with my long-planned bike ride while I was still able, raising money for Alzheimer's Research along the way, her reply was unequivocal. 'Go, Chris. Do it. Before it's too late.'

Forward march!

Never one to shy away from a challenge, I won't

19

let a little thing like early-onset Alzheimer's get in my way. Every mile I notched up on my tracker was a mile closer to home, and to her. I'd been on the road since 4 a.m. and my left knee was niggling, but it wasn't a showstopper and I hoped it would square itself away in time. Yes, I'd been far too cavalier and made a stupid error – due in part to my general confusion and increasing memory lapses – but, hey, that was life.

I had to stop thinking. Thinking's dangerous with me. It was time to forge on and find somewhere for Shirley, my trailer and me. Then I'd pitch my one-man tent, put some calories and my supplements inside me, and try to get some zeds. There'd be no secure campsite with electric fencing for me that night, no Wi-Fi via which to check in with Vicks.

I only hoped I wouldn't get eaten alive. Not that I'd make much of a meal. The regulation SA80 rifle I'd carried as an Army commando for most of my military career had been replaced with bear deterrents including bangers and spray. The instructions on the can didn't exactly instil confidence: *Use to deter an aggressive or charging bear. The recommended minimum distance between user and bear should be 25 feet. Using the spray improperly can have undesirable effects ... and may actually attract bears.*

Brilliant.

'If a grizzly charges us, you're on your own, Shirley,' I told my trusty steed as I hurriedly pegged down my tent next to her. 'Out here, it's every idiot for themselves.' Her Union flag was looking bedraggled and her burgundy paintwork and wheel guards were splattered with mud, so I vowed to give her a bit of spit and polish before we set off again in the chill of the dawn.

As the light leached from the Canadian sky and the wilderness creatures began their nightly cacophony, I crawled inside my nylon billet and pulled my mess tin and army rations out of the panniers that made up part of my seventy-kilo kit. I didn't dare risk cooking up anything that might attract unwelcome visitors so I'd have to eat cold. It would be a bar of chocolate and a cheese and ham sarnie for me.

Scoffing my scran by torchlight, I welcomed the sensation of food in my belly – however un-appetising. My rumbling tummy reminded me of being permanently hungry at our freezing-cold council house in Bowdon Vale on the outskirts of Manchester, where I grew up with my brother, Anthony, and two sisters, Ange and Lizzie.

Now Anthony, or Tony as I called him, was forty-three years old and in a nursing home being drip-fed from a tube. I had no idea how much longer it would be before I was in a similar state. I had to stop dwelling on that kind of thing, though. It didn't help anyone. Sure, one day this cruel disease was going to bite me on the arse, but for now I was fit and well and making this once-in-a-lifetime adventure for a great cause.

Besides, I had a lot to live up to. As David Cameron announced to the nation shortly before I set off (yes, that's right, the British Prime Minis-ter!), I had his 'absolute backing' for my 'mam-moth challenge' and 'daunting, once-in-a-lifetime journey'. Speaking in response to an email Vicks

21

had sent to Downing Street to inform him of my challenge, the PM added that I was 'a great example of someone who, when faced with a difficult diagnosis, has shown extraordinary grit and determination to overcome his circumstances and ensure that future generations can benefit from potentially life-saving research'.

How about that, then? Not bad for a scab-kneed kid from the wrong side of the tracks.

So, it was time for this scab-kneed civvy to get his head down and have some shut-eye. It would be another 4 a.m. start and there was some difficult terrain looming up ahead of me, not least the Rocky Mountains – which I'd have to cross twice.

'Night, Shirley,' I called into the darkness, switching off my head torch. As I slid into my sleeping bag, having checked it carefully for critters, I heard a rustling noise somewhere close by and then something screeched demonically. Snapping my torch back on and holding my breath, I listened some more but there was only silence. Wriggling further in and zipping myself right up to the neck, I turned off the light and tried not to dwell on the fact that if I was attacked my cries for help would go unheard in the wilderness.

If in doubt – kip.

1

'It is good to have an end to journey toward; but it is the journey that matters most in the end.'
ERNEST HEMINGWAY

Dementia Adventure Diary, Spring 2015, Brize Norton, Oxfordshire, England

I'd never been much of a cyclist and was always keener on running and playing football. I'm more of a general all-rounder who's done the odd sporting event here and there – including one of the biggies, the Mount Everest Marathon, which was a little cheeky in parts.

Although cycling had never appealed to me before, like most people I enjoyed cheering on Team GB at the Velodrome in the Olympics. My perspective changed however when I watched Scottish adventurer Mark Beaumont on his televised 13,000-mile bike ride from Anchorage, Alaska, to southern Argentina in 2010. Mark had already smashed the world record for cycling round the world in 194 days, but his quest to cycle the longest mountain range on earth *and* climb its two highest peaks in the Rockies and the Andes along the way planted a seed in my addled brain and I was inspired.

Like Mark, I wanted to achieve something extraordinary – both for myself and to raise as much money as I could for the two charities that will undoubtedly end up helping me, and my family. I couldn't think of a more fitting end to my military career. The work funded by Alzheimer's Research will probably be too late to make any difference to my life, but it might just save my kids, who are living under threat of the same fate. And ABF The Soldiers' Charity, formerly known as the Army Benevolent Fund, does a grand job of looking after those families whose military breadwinners have fallen on hard times, so I hoped to raise a few thousand quid for them too.

My initial plan was to complete my Dementia Adventure with Neil Deadman, my best mate from primary school, but he had to drop out at the last minute. It was undoubtedly one of his smartest moves, because he'd have never kept up with me.

Determined to press on regardless, and with Vicky's blessing, I decided to be as self-sufficient as possible while pushing myself to the limit. For a journey I expected to take a full year, starting in the spring of 2015, I'd be enduring everything from the bitter North American winter to the scorching deserts of Arizona and California on what was very much a personal challenge. I suppose it was also a way of giving myself time to get my head around a future where I'd never be self-sufficient again.

The sad news is that, in terms of my disease, I am far from alone. Quite apart from the rare genetic blight that affects my own family, every minute of every hour someone new in the world is diagnosed with one or other type of this disease that gradually kills off brain cells. One in three of us over the age of sixty-five will have to learn to live with dementia, and two-thirds of those are women – who are twice as likely to develop it in their sixties as they are breast cancer. This represents nothing short of an epidemic and one of the biggest medical challenges the world faces. Alzheimer's is one of the most common causes of dementia. It's a ticking time bomb and one of the world's leading causes of death.

As yet, there is no cure.

In embarking on my solo charity bike ride, I knew I'd be testing my mental and physical endurance to the max. So it was important that I make the route as simple as possible. I chose North America because I'd been there several times before and I knew and liked the place. It's English-speaking, its people are friendly and it offers a diverse range of landscapes, history and culture. I hoped that, once across the Atlantic, my small wheel tracks would make a big enough impression to raise awareness and secure at least £40,000 for the cause. I'm not sure why I settled on that target figure – maybe because I'd be forty at the end of the ride – but I didn't honestly know if I'd raise a penny or if anyone would be interested in following my progress. I was staggered then when we topped £20,000 within twenty-four hours of Vicky setting up my website in March, especially as I hadn't cycled a single mile yet. My online response was: 'Wow! Many thanks for all the support, everyone!'

Seated at our map-covered dining table, Vicks and I drank umpteen cups of Rosy Lee as we worked out the best route to take me across seven provinces in Canada and through twenty-six US states, following the coastline as much as possible. We began by working out a 14,000-mile route from Ontario but then I added a cheeky 2,000 miles by starting in Halifax, Nova Scotia, on the east coast of Canada. Neil Deadman's comment on my upgrade was, 'Nova Scotia? Another little detour! Since when was 14,000 miles not enough?!'

Then I'd pedal all the way across Canada through Manitoba, Saskatchewan, Alberta, British Columbia and the Yukon to Anchorage on the north-west coast of Alaska, before retracing some of my tracks to get back on the road south all the way through Washington, Oregon, Nevada, California, Arizona and New Mexico. I then hoped to ride across the full width of the southern US through Texas, Louisiana, Alabama, Mississippi and Georgia to the Florida Keys, and up the east coast through the Carolinas, Virginia, Maryland, Delaware, New Jersey and Pennsylvania to New York, before returning to my starting point via Connecticut and Maine.

'I plan to travel light and move fast,' I told Vicky from the outset, reciting the mantra I'd adopted for my ride. Although I'd pedalled round Yorkshire with some disabled veterans for the Help for Heroes charity, the furthest I'd ever cycled in a single day before was thirty-eight miles through the Cotswold countryside from my home to Cirencester and back – and then only after I'd bought the rig for this trip. As with much of my life, I was just going to go for it. Based on my

26

previous and limited experience, I estimated that I could comfortably ride forty miles a day. With that in mind, Vicky and I had to work out roughly how long each leg would take me depending on distance, climate and terrain, and then figure out where I'd end up during the most extreme seasons of summer and winter.

Vicks also logged my 5ft 7ins height and eleven stone (70 kg) weight into various charts and painstakingly worked out a crib sheet for my dietary needs. She reckoned that I'd need at least six thousand calories and six litres of water per day, all of which we tried to budget for accordingly. I'd carry Army ration packs but would only use them in emergencies, buying cheap high-carbohydrate food along the way.

'Pizza and burgers every day? What's not to like?' I told her with a grin.

We suspected that I might have problems finding accommodation in some of the more remote areas, so I'd try to sleep in my tent as much as possible for ease and in order to keep costs down. I'd only check into a motel once a week for rest days and a chance to wash off the sweat and the dirt.

Once the route was sorted, it was time to get myself kitted out. I wrote a long list of the equipment I thought I should carry but in retrospect I was largely clueless when it came to cycling. Fortunately, I'd paid close attention to the rig Mark Beaumont took around the Americas and I asked a few bike-mad mates for their advice. With a rough idea of what I might need, I went into a local cycling shop called Mountain Mania and announced, 'I'm about to do a 16,000-mile ride around North America but I know bugger all about bikes. Can you help me?' They clearly thought I was suffering from some sort of mania myself, but were incredibly patient nevertheless as I went back and forth to discuss the permutations.

With their help, I finally settled on my Surly Long Haul Disc Trucker equipped with a Brooks saddle, Schwalbe tyres, Voyager One trailer, Supernova lights and six panniers. It wasn't cheap – that little lot came to just short of £4,000, and that was with the discount they kindly offered me. As my tent was going to be my primary home for a year I chose a one-man Hilleberg, which set me back an additional £600. Then I needed a hammock, roll mat, sleeping bag, pillow, air horn, cooking equipment, my ration packs, water carriers, medical pack, tools and spares. I'd require breathable lightweight all-weather clothing, eye and sun protection, a helmet, mobile phone, chargers, and various navigation devices. With its panniers full, my bike and body weight totalled a shocking twenty stone, or 138 kg.

So much for my 'fast and light' mantra.

'Bloody hell, Gurkha,' one of my mates quipped, calling me by my military nickname. 'You're certainly going to be living up to your name with that lot on board!'

I didn't have a clue how to go about seeking sponsorship for my ride and I didn't imagine that anyone would want to sponsor me anyway, so I went ahead and coughed up for almost everything out of my recent Army pay-off. Alzheimer's Research agreed to pay for my return flights, which helped enormously, and some stoic members of our local Rotary Club cycled the 150-mile Oxfordshire Ridgeway over a weekend to raise £1,000 towards my costs. A few of the old boys were so sore they couldn't even sit down afterwards, but I jokingly called them 'lazy swine' and reminded them that I'd be aiming to cycle that kind of distance on a good day.

A couple of friends generously shelled out for a GoPro camera and my Yellowbrick two-way satellite tracking device – the type originally designed for yachtsmen far from any phone signal, and from which I could also send messages and texts. It would 'ping' my precise latitude and longitude every few miles and plot them on an interactive map that Vicky and others could follow.

From then on in, though, it was all down to me.

No pressure then.

My biggest problem after I'd forked out more than half of my military gratuity was working out exactly how to balance all my kit on the bike. Each pannier needed to weigh the same as its counterpart on the opposite side or it would pull me over, especially in high winds. Setting off on my first few training rides with my feet clipped into the pedals as advised, I wobbled like a toddler without stabilisers and almost came a cropper. It took me a bit of practice but I finally worked out the best way to manage the weight.

Not that I did much more preparation than that, to be honest. Even though I'd never undertaken anything as challenging as this before, I figured that although the first few weeks would be tough I'd be all right once my legs acquired muscle memory. I'd done quite a few endurance runs in the past and was confident I'd be able to pull it off physically. My only worry was how to keep going day after day and break through the pain barriers, the 'wall' that athletes refer to. I just hoped my body would adapt.

Because I'm not at all switched on when it comes to modern technology, Vicky sorted out all the online stuff for me, including setting up my Yellowbrick account, the social media pages that would become the diary of my trip, and our Long Cycle Round website where people could follow my progress via the links and on Google Maps. Then she organised a Just Giving page where friends could donate money towards my target.

Alzheimer's Research was really supportive from the start and created a video promoting my ride. In it, chief executive Hilary Evans said: 'Chris's fundraising efforts mean a huge amount to Alzheimer's Research UK. It's fantastic to have someone in his position who's been diagnosed with Alzheimer's at such an early age and who has turned around this diagnosis – which is devastating for Chris and his family – into such a positive, showing that there is hope; and Chris has that hope in research... Raising this money is going to help us find those treatments and prevent the next generation of people having to live with Alzheimer's.'

Robin Bacon of ABF The Soldiers' Charity added, 'Chris's fundraising is having a significant impact because he has such an interesting story... It encourages people to think, "My goodness, if he can do it then he deserves some support."'

I was almost set to go when there was a last-minute glitch with our carefully executed plans. Booking the flights, we discovered that flying to Nova Scotia would be prohibitively expensive (the thieving weasels!) so we had to settle on Toronto, Ontario, as my starting point instead. If I had the time I still hoped to make it up to Halifax and back at the end of my ride, just so that I could say I reached all four corners of that vast continent and crossed them off my bucket list.

With my airline tickets purchased, all that was left to do was sort insurance and make sure Vicks had everything she needed to follow me on a phone and our two laptops. Then it was time to pack my freshly washed smalls – although only a couple of pairs because I didn't expect to wear them often under my skin-tight Lycra.

'Don't get overtired, Chris,' she began to warn me as her nerves kicked in. 'You know that only makes your symptoms worse. And keep taking your vitamins. Listen to your body whenever it tells you to take a break. You'll make a potentially fatal decision if you're not thinking clearly.'

I gave her my best 'get-out-of-shit-quick' smile and told her cheerfully, 'Stand at ease, babes. Loads of people do this kind of thing and they all make it home in one piece.'

Her face darkened for a moment. 'I know, Chris,' she said quietly. 'But none of them have terminal Alzheimer's...'

Fair comment.

The worst moment was undoubtedly saying goodbye to her and my family for what I knew would be the best part of a year. Vicky and I curled up in bed that last night clinging to each other like a couple of shipwrecked mariners. She handed me three envelopes and told me to pack them away for the journey. 'Only open them when you need a hug,' she instructed firmly.

I was really looking forward to my trip but secretly worried that I was being selfish leaving her on her own for a year, especially when we had so little time left together. And then there was Dexter to consider. My departure came almost three months to the day since our precious boy was born, and although I had two teenage children from a previous marriage, being a father once again with this diagnosis hanging over me (and them) felt even more significant somehow.

I knew I hadn't been a great dad to my older kids, Natalie and Marcus, but that was due in part to geography – they lived with their mother in Norway and I'd been 'Army barmy' in far-flung countries for most of their young lives. The saddest thing now was that I probably wouldn't have the time to make it up to them, or give them the kind of joyful memories I never had of my own father.

In fact, I only have two clear recollections of my dad, and neither of them was great. The first must have been in about 1979, when I was three years old. The man I can barely remember wandered into the living room where I was sitting on the sofa with my mum Dorothy, watching television, and he made a strange sound. We looked up and I noticed that he was foaming at the mouth. In his hand was a bottle of washing-up liquid that he'd been drinking from as if it were juice.

'No, John!' cried Mum, jumping up to grab it. He struggled with her and was clearly upset. Later that day, two strange men arrived at our house and took him away. Dad shouted a bit at first and then he was gone, led from the room like a scolded child. I didn't see him again for at least another year and no mention of him was made. Because none of the doctors knew exactly what was wrong with him to begin with, he ended up being sent to a mental hospital.

My second memory of Dad was the time my brother Tony and I were taken to visit him there. I don't think my older sister Angie came with us then and my little sister Lizzie would have been too young. Parkside Hospital in Macclesfield was a forbidding red-brick building set in several acres of grounds. I remember it smelled overwhelmingly of disinfectant. The wing we were ushered into had an unusual domed roof, like one of the barracks I was later based in. We found Dad drugged up and gone in the head, curled up on his bed like a baby. He was on what we referred to as 'Planet Pluto' and being fed through a tube. God knows what medication they gave dementia patients back then. He didn't know or recognise us, so Tony and I wandered off to play table tennis in a nearby room as Mum sat, pale and silent, by his side.

Less than a year later, on 1 November 1981, my father was gone. I was almost six years old when he passed away. John Richard Graham, a happy-go-lucky and famously unpunctual mechanical fitter who'd once held down a good job at an instrument gauge factory and been happily married with four children, died alone in that loony bin at forty-two. Friends of the family said he looked twice that age by the end. My mother received a phone call at home to tell her that he'd died and she called us kids in from playing outside to tell us. Not that I remember much more than that. What I do remember is that Dad was never talked about and there were no photographs of him on display. It was as if he'd been erased. Mum was devastated but even she had to smile at his cremation because, after years of her telling him he'd be late to his own funeral, he was.

His death certificate states that he died of bronchopneumonia and pre-senile dementia, although for a long time Mum and the family were told variously that he had 'water on the brain' or a degenerative neurological condition called Huntington's chorea. Either way, she never got over it and – in many ways – neither did any of us.

None of us knew back then that his true cause of death was a rare genetic mutation labelled 'PSEN1' that cruelly gives Alzheimer's disease to random members of our family at a premature age. PSEN stands for Presenilin, because it causes Alzheimer's at a 'pre-senile' age. With a faulty PSEN gene, a damaging protein builds up in the brain causing first the connections between brain cells and then the cells themselves to die, which leads to progressive mental deterioration. This build-up happens in all Alzheimer's cases, but with our faulty gene, it happens decades earlier.

My grandfather had died of early-onset Alzheimer's aged forty-six, although nobody would admit to anything as shaming as an inherited illness at the time. Instead, they claimed he had 'shell shock' after his experiences in the Second World War, which was a common excuse for any unexplained neurological condition along with being 'doolally' or 'feeble-minded', or 'going funny in the head'. When my aunt Thelma died of dementia before the age of forty, our relatives still didn't appear to make any connection and blamed her so-called 'mental confusion' on a beating she'd allegedly received. By the time my father died of it, any possible connection was either covered up or ignored.

Thankfully, since the 1980s, scientists understand so much more about the condition and especially about our rare genetic mutation, which occurs on chromosome number 14 in human DNA. They know, for example, that the average age at onset of symptoms is thirty-seven and the average age of death is forty-four. They also know that fifty per cent of people in an affected family will develop the disease. What they don't know is what switches the gene on and – more importantly – how to repair it.

I was thirty-three and a father of two when my brother Tony was finally diagnosed at the age of thirty-seven. Having eventually been told that I too might be affected, I decided to have the test. That's when I received the shocking news that I did carry the mutant gene, although I had no obvious symptoms yet. It was four years later and not long after I met Vicky that I discovered that the bomb inside me had detonated.

With a new baby on the way, I became even more determined to do all I could to try to beat my new enemy – the rogue mutation that cruelly threatened to take me away from everyone I'd ever loved. It would quite literally be a fight to the death, and my endurance ride around North America would be my first major bout.

Fix bayonets!

The good news was that I had massive support back home – not just Vicks but my sisters and all my old school chums and military colleagues or, as we jokingly referred to each other, 'shipmates'. All of them encouraged me privately and publicly. The day I flew to Canada, my friend Neil posted a typical comment on Facebook: 'My best mate Chris Graham is off to Toronto this morning to start his epic 16,000 mile charity bike ride. Very proud of him. Good luck brother. You'll smash it, I'm sure!'

With friends like that, I couldn't possibly give up. Failure was not an option for this soldier.

On the day I left the UK, I fastened my seat-belt, took a deep breath, and sat back as the Iceland Air plane flying me across the Atlantic Ocean via Reykjavik began to speed along the runway. At last it lifted off, taking me skywards to my big adventure and the first leg of my long journey through dementia.

If in doubt – keep moving.

2

'Life is like riding a bicycle. To keep your balance, you have to keep moving.'

ALBERT EINSTEIN

Dementia Adventure Diary, 26 April 2015, Brighton, Ontario, Canada

I plugged in my earphones and turned on my iPhone so that I could hear Vicky's lovely voice in my head. Then, early that frosty April, I headed west out of Toronto on Highway 2 for the beginning of my madcap adventure. Next stop, Anchorage.

With a start in Nova Scotia unaffordable, I was setting off instead from the house of my mate Dean Stokes – 'Stokesie' – and his wife Nicole. In a random phone call I'd asked the former sergeant major if I could stay a few nights and if he could pick me up, along with my bike and all my kit, from the airport. 'I've only got a Honda Accord!' he protested. But he found a larger vehicle and not only met me but took fantastic care of me before my trip, promising to do the same after – if I made it back in one piece. Stokesie even agreed to accompany me on my first day's ride to get me accustomed to Canadian roads.

'I can't believe you're finally doing this!' Vicky cried excitedly down the phone, as Nicole waved us off that first morning. I heard Dexter gurgling away in the background and could just picture our infant son, snotty-nosed and red-eyed, resting on his mother's hip. It would have been about four in the morning in the UK and I'm sure Vicky was utterly cream crackered, but she'd never let me hear that in our daily calls.

The girlfriend I ended up dubbing my 'long-haired colonel' had no idea yet what she was in for. Self-sufficiency had always been my objective on this unsupported expedition of mine, but that probably wasn't realistic with the state of my colander brain. It's possible that I could have completed the ride without her guidance but it would have been that much more difficult and taken me a whole lot longer. To be honest, I think I'd still be on the road now!

Once Vicks was satisfied that I was on my way that first day and wouldn't need her further guidance or encouragement for a while, she finally relented and went to bed. Knowing her, she'd only allow herself a few hours' sleep before getting up again to check on me. I think it reassured her to know that forty-six-year-old Dean, a former member of the Parachute Regiment and chief instructor of jungle training who'd worked alongside me in Sierra Leone, was with me for the first day. And that we'd gone on a sixteen-mile test run together to make sure that everything on 'Shirley' was working properly after she'd been rebuilt by the staff at Dean's local bike shop, Tri&Run in Trenton, having been dismantled for the flight. Visibility was vitally important on the kinds of roads I'd be travelling on, so over a bacon butty after our trial, Dean and I agreed that I should add an extra light to my trailer.

Back we went to the bike shop, where Sandy the owner and Craig the mechanic kindly sorted me out. As we were leaving, I told them, 'Thanks guys. I'll come and see you on my way home for a cup of tea and tell you all about it.'

'We'll hold you to that!' they replied, with a thumbs up.

I'd been so relieved when Dean offered to ride alongside me to begin with – well, I say 'alongside', but he'd be the first to admit that he found it a struggle to keep up with me. And I was hauling a total weight of twenty stone!

'That's when I appreciated just how fit Chris was,' he said later. 'I was always behind him and finding it very hard going in the gusty winds, especially once we left sea level and started to climb north. Twice, when we stopped, I fell off my bike with my feet still clipped into the pedals and hurt myself – but mostly my pride.'

Mercifully for Dean, he received a call from Nicole some six miles into the day. A Canadian medic, she rang to tell him she'd been scrambled to Nepal to help victims of the recent earthquake. She wanted him to help her get ready so he had to turn around and go home. I have to admit that was a bit of a scary moment for me. 'You're leaving me – on my own?' I asked, saucer-eyed.

'Sorry, but Nicole needs me,' he replied, shrugging. 'Chin up, mate. You've only got another 15,990 miles to go. See you in a year!'

I watched him disappear and took a deep breath. He was right. This was really happening. I'd have to get used to being on my own so now was as good a time as any to start. Just before setting off again I switched to the specially selected music playlist on my phone. I'd downloaded about fifty favourite songs, most of which were uplifting or had a strong beat to cycle to. I had to laugh when the first number that came up was 'Tears and Rain' from the album *Back to Bedlam* by James Blunt. I was surely headed for a kind of Bedlam one day, and as freezing rain started to lash my face, making my eyes water, this seemed the perfect tune.

How I wish I could walk through the doors of my mind. Hold memory close at hand, the former cavalry officer sang. I doubted there were that many doors in my brain, but I knew I'd be holding my memories close as the prospect of a year largely alone with my mind stretched ahead of me.

As I settled into the ride and tried to adjust my position so that my back and legs felt more comfortable, I zoned into the music playing in my ears and was grateful that the first phase of my journey would be relatively straightforward, following well-signposted routes that shouldn't tax my memory too much. Truth was, I was finding it increasingly difficult to remember things and whenever I underwent further cognitive tests at the various hospitals where I was being monitored, I didn't fare that well.

My old schoolmate Neil came with me on one early assessment in London and watched as I was given three things to remember. By the time I'd got to the third, the first one had flown right out of my mind. In the next task, the doctor in charge asked me to identify different objects. 'What's this?' he asked, holding up a card with a photograph on it.

'A shovel,' I replied confidently.

'Good, Chris. Now give me a sentence that has that word in it.'

Smiling impishly I suggested, 'Sticks like shit to a shovel?' The doc grinned back at me, but five minutes later when he showed me the same photograph, I struggled to recall what it was and I couldn't for the life of me remember the sentence I'd given him moments before.

Even though I was clearly having difficulty, when I told Professor Nick Fox – the man in charge – about my planned charity bike ride later on, he was all for me going ahead with it. 'You have my blessing, Chris,' he told me. 'My advice to you is to do as much as you can, while you still can.'

I've always been terrible with directions, which isn't altogether helpful when cycling around North America on your own, but I'd assured Vicks I'd be able to rely on my GPS navigation and various tracking devices on which I could plot my daily route. What we didn't appreciate until I set off was that this would mean I'd be constantly looking down at my phone or satnav whilst on the road, which wasn't the safest option. Plus most of my kit was dependent on good mobile phone service and working batteries in places without access to either.

Chris Graham – mini genius.

From those earliest days of my ride, the dangers were apparent because it was vital to look where I was going, especially once I had my first encounters with what would come to represent my greatest risk. These were huge trucks whose drivers were sitting eight feet or more above the road, playing music or chatting away on their GB radios, barely aware of lesser mortals such as me. I'd first spot them looming up behind me in my wing mirrors, reminding me of that moment in *Jurassic Park* when the Tyrannosaurus Rex closes in on the Jeep as its hapless driver sees the etched message in his mirror which reads, *Objects in the Mirror are Closer than they Appear.* I knew just how they felt as these forty-ton giants bore down on me.

With only a few seconds to decide what best to do as they came dangerously close, I'd either turn Shirley onto the hard shoulder and risk falling off and injuring myself, or try to stick it out on the tarmac only to be blown off course by their powerful slipstreams. The Canadian roads were generally in good condition, with tarmac and some gravel but – with the recent snows – the hard shoulders were clogged with salt and gravel that had been repeatedly ploughed there throughout the winter.

This left just a few narrow strips that I could only ride on if I gripped the handlebars so tightly that my fingers cramped and my palms bruised, even through padded gloves. It was like being in a permanent press-up position. Plus my hands got so cold that they went numb and I couldn't operate the brakes after a while. Whenever I stopped and tried to stretch my fingers out, they'd click into position like ratchets.

Each time I wobbled back onto the carriageway

to give my hands a break or avoid another mini-iceberg, passing truck drivers would sound their klaxons just as they were about to crush me, the shock of which could make me jump right out of my saddle. I ended up with scabby elbows and legs as well as some impressive bruises on my *glutei maximi* – buttocks to you and me.

Not that I was a stranger to bruises and scuffed knees. My two sisters and most of my school-mates would confirm that I was always getting into scrapes. And I started young. In 1978, when I was just eighteen months old, I pulled the table-cloth and a freshly made pot of tea off the kitchen table, tipping it all over me. I ended up with third-degree burns on my right arm.

My mum's best friend Joan Hill was there that afternoon and remembers it well. 'Chris was badly scalded and I went with Dorothy straight away to Pendlebury Children's Hospital where he was kept in for three days. He ended up having to have a series of skin grafts but they didn't really help with the scarring. His injuries were so serious that medical staff and social ser-vices questioned his mother on suspicion of inflicting them. It was a horrible time.'

Poor Mum. As if she didn't have enough on her plate with my newborn sister Lizzie and Dad already starting to be forgetful. I don't remember anything about the teapot incident but I've lived with the scars my whole life – they're still visible from my shoulder to the inside of my elbow, plus I have a hairless rectangle on my leg where the skin graft came from.

In another infamous escapade when I was eight,

I somehow got myself stuck in the wooden headboard of the bunk bed I shared with Lizzie – known as 'our kid' – in our three-bedroomed terraced council house in Eaton Road, Bowdon Vale. I've always been restless and had too much energy – even when asleep. After another night of constant motion, in which I was probably reenacting my favourite scene in *Superman II* when Clark Kent rescues a boy from Niagara Falls, I somehow managed to wedge myself through a six-inch gap and ended up trapped around my waist. I was shouting 'Help!' for ages before Mum heard me at around 2 a.m., and assumed I was having a nightmare until she came into the bedroom and found me. She called an ambulance and a policeman arrived also. But in typical no-nonsense fashion, she insisted they didn't cut into the headboard to get me out because she couldn't afford to replace it.

They struggled to no avail for almost an hour to pull me clear and then some bright spark came up with the idea of slathering me in butter. The story made the local newspapers, with headlines like 'Bedtime story' and 'Butter frees bed prisoner'. One article described me as 'mischievous' and said I thought the whole 'adventure' was 'smashing'. I'm sure my mother was furious at the disruption I caused her and the entire street, but especially at the loss of a perfectly good pound of butter.

She was the kind of mother who did the best she could for us in very difficult circumstances, but she was never a loveydovey sort of mum. She was too busy struggling to hold down three jobs, including her main one as the caretaker of a local primary school. She also suffered from depression when my dad was sent to the mental hospital, and especially after he died.

I never told any of my friends what had really happened to my dad and I never told anyone how badly it affected my mum. Falling in with a Graham family trait, I didn't speak about it at all. Neil Deadman and my other friends at school knew only that I didn't have a father. As Neil said, 'We would never have known things were so bad at home. Chris was always so happy-go-lucky and never one to dwell on things. He wasn't the type to get down or angry. His brother Tony was a bit deeper and more thoughtful, but Chris wasn't like that at all.'

In fact I was so defiantly cheerful that Neil's dad apparently wanted to adopt me. He played football with us and told his wife that I was such a great kid he'd gladly have taken me in. I don't think he felt sorry for me exactly, but he appreciated early on that I'd benefit from a father figure, especially someone who'd encourage me in sport. I loved football and, being nippy with a good engine, I was picked for school teams in the Trafford area and for a local boys' club. From as young as I can recall, I was a big Manchester United fan thanks to my brother Tony, who was old enough to remember that Dad had been a keen supporter.

Once a Red, always a Red 'til the day you die, we say. I still can't quite get over the fact that my old mate Neil Deadman supports Manchester City, the dirty blue nose.

My favourite United player was Bryan Robson who was loyal, a clever team player, selfless, down to earth and an all-round top bloke (not to mention a future England captain). As a kid, I could never afford to attend any of the matches to see him playing in person, so I'd watch him on the telly instead. The first live football match I went to was actually a rival Man City game – and only because Neil's dad treated us (but don't tell my fellow United fans).

The good thing about living in 'Soapy Town' – the local nickname for Bowdon Vale, because of how much washing was taken in for the well-off neighbours up the hill – is that nobody else had much money either, so we didn't especially stick out. I'm sure we weren't the only family who had to turn out the lights and hide whenever creditors came knocking at the door or the sinister-looking television licence van circled the neighbourhood. Nor were we the only kids locked out of our house after school until Mum came home, hanging around in all weathers or sponging off friends until her shift ended. It was only when I went to a different secondary school to many of my mates that I came to the uncomfortable realisation that I was quite underprivileged.

Luck wasn't always against me, though. I remember playing on a building site once and coming across a five-pound note. I could hardly believe it when I spotted it poking out of the rubble. Excitedly, I ran straight home and gave it to my mum. I was hero of the hour until I got into trouble with the busies – the police – soon afterwards for pinching a bottle of milk from a float. It wasn't the first – or the last – time I nicked things, but in fairness to me it was usually some orange juice from a doorstep for my little sister Lizzie.

We Graham children were poor enough to qualify for free school dinners, which was definitely the best thing about being deprived. I ate shit loads at every sitting and then scoffed all the leftovers from others' plates. I was hungry my entire childhood and Vicks will tell you that not much has changed. 'I've never known anyone so small eat so much,' is her frequent complaint. There were a few posh kids at school who complained about the quality of the food we were served but I thought it just fine and dandy. After grabbing a piece of toast or a mouthful of cereal for breakfast each morning I'd be out of the door like a cork out of a bottle, so by dinnertime I was gagging for a drink and always half-starved.

When I got home in the evenings Mum would sit the four of us either side of a rough picnic bench-cum-table in our kitchen and dish up something like a hotpot made with cheap cuts, and she always prepared a Sunday dinner. There might not have been much of it to go around but it was tasty. We couldn't fail to notice that she often skipped her tea so that we could eat, and stood watching us instead with a cup of coffee and a cigarette. More often than not, my tea would be something out of a tin – spaghetti hoops or baked beans – because I didn't make it home in time. Following in my big brother Tony's footsteps, I virtually did as I pleased once Dad had died, and became a bit of a brat.

Instead of doing my homework or helping with the chores, I'd kick a football around with Neil Deadman, Craig Calder, Kevin Molson or John

Ollier. We lads also messed about around the Bollin River for hours, creating dens and making rafts. My happiest childhood memories are undoubtedly of those long hot summers in Bowdon Vale when there was no school and the days seemed to last forever while we ran wild in Bollin Woods. With or without school to go to, most nights I'd arrive back home long after dark, filthy, wet and cold. Mum would lose her temper and give me a clip round the ear before putting me on short rations and grounding me for a day or two.

Ange also took a lot of stick because she was the eldest girl, but my recollection is that she and Lizzie never seemed to get it in the neck as much as we boys because Mum found girls easier to control. My sisters would argue that I was allowed to get away with murder thanks to my baby face. Lizzie even dubbed me the 'golden child'. She said that whenever I was naughty, they'd all be punished for it. 'Mum would line us up on the settee and march up and down like a sergeant major, demanding to know who was responsible. Angie and I would glare at Chris, who'd smile angelically and never say a word, and we'd all be grounded. He was dreadful like that!'

Lizzie tagged along with me whenever she could, and I rarely turned her back. I knew what it felt like to be excluded every time my big brother told me to bugger off and stop bothering him and his mates. I'd sit her in an old tyre in the middle of our latest raft before me and my pals would push off from the bank and head down river. Often, we'd make it all the way to Dunham before the thing broke apart. Lizzie and I would have to walk the hour back home, dripping wet. If ever she complained she was hungry or thirsty, I'd nip into a shop or jump over a garden wall to pinch her something to eat or drink.

One day I persuaded my mates we should camp out in the woods all night. I knew Lizzie would have tried to join us so I didn't even tell her. While Mum was working at the old people's home, I sneaked to the cupboard and pulled out some clean bed linen. Then I took some food from the kitchen and carried it down to our secret hideaway. When everyone in the house was asleep, I jumped out of the bedroom window, slid down the drainpipe and ran to the woods. Sadly, all my friends lost their bottle and not one of them showed up, but – just in case they did – I stuck it out until dawn, watching the sun creep over the horizon with a childish sense of wonder and excitement while shivering with cold.

It wasn't much warmer at home, where we couldn't afford to have the heating on. There was a three-bar gas fire in the lounge fed by a fifty-pence meter, but it was rarely on and then only one bar worked. As a consequence, the house was damp and the wood on the window frames was so rotten that I could push my fingers right through it. We only had a bath once a week, which wasn't that unusual in the Vale, but after Dad died that became a problem because I frequently wet the bed. I was so ashamed I wouldn't tell Mum and would sleep somewhere else rather than on the damp patch. I was even more embarrassed when I realised that I smelled of wee.

I also became sore with the constant wetness

and chafing and frequently asked to be excused in class to use the loo. The next thing I knew, Mum took me to a doctor about my 'weak bladder' and he put me in hospital. I must have been eight years old when I was medically circumcised, and it really hurt. I also hated having to stay on the ward for a few days afterwards, but Mum bought me some A-Team men and a box of Lego to cheer me up, which made my sisters insanely jealous. I was sent home with my new toys a day or so later. But I still wet the bed.

Needless to say, I was scruffy and smelly. When I invited the first girl I ever had a crush on round to my house, she was horrified at where we lived and the state I was in. After calling me a 'tramp' she left. I never invited anyone else back after that.

My mother would have been mortified had she heard. Like most of the women on our estate, she may have been stony broke but she was still proud and managed the best she could in near impossible circumstances. She was embarrassed anytime we were offered charity and horrified when Tony, Angie and I appeared on the front page of the *Altrincham Messenger* in an article about 'underprivileged children' being taken to a local pantomime for free. When Lizzie was born on the day of the Queen's Jubilee in June 1977, there was a street party in nearby Bollin Avenue. Feeling the baby coming on and knowing she'd be out of action for a few days, Mum went home and scrubbed the kitchen floor thoroughly before asking her friend Joan to drive her to the hospital.

Lizzie is a sweetheart and has always been

devoted to me. I think of us more as twins than siblings separated by eighteen months. Ange is three years older than me and, without doubt, the smartest one in the family. She even passed her eleven-plus examination and earned her place in the local grammar school, a first for our family. Mum was dead proud. By contrast, I was as thick as two planks and all I really cared about at school was PE – though I did like history and geography too, especially the idea of a big wide world out there just waiting to be explored. When the Falklands War began in 1982 I was six years old and soon became transfixed by the idea of becoming a soldier and fighting for the Queen.

It was my dream to make my country – and my mother – proud.

I must have been eight when Mum started dating her boss Eric, a man who'd been married before and had children. They worked together at a local factory that made clothing for the Girl Guides. Widowed, alone and without a proverbial pot to piss in, my mother probably hoped Eric would save us all from destitution. Before we had time to get used to the idea of them dating, he'd moved in and assumed the role of father figure, especially over Tony and me who were out of control.

When Mum and Eric married at the local registry office a year later, Ange and Lizzie were specially dressed in matching purple suits from a local shop called Tammy Girl. Tony and I were badgered into washing our faces, slicking down our hair, and putting on a shirt and tie. Neither of us ever took to Eric, though, and it can't have been long afterwards that I started to rebel, yelling at him, 'You can't tell me what to do. You're not my dad!'

I didn't really remember my father, but I had a childishly nostalgic notion of the man I thought he was and stubbornly refused to accept the new person in our mother's affections. In retrospect, Eric wasn't a bad bloke – he never hit us or shouted, anyway – but Mum seemed to change overnight. She became far more subdued and encouraged him to discipline us, as she no longer could. I resented that, but I was probably just being immature.

It was undoubtedly thanks to the financial security that Eric brought to our household that I was given my best ever Christmas present. Mum had always made a fuss of us at that time of year even before Eric came on the scene. I don't know how she managed it but we'd come down in the morning and there'd be loads of presents under the tree. Angie recalled, 'She bought everything from Brian the catalogue man, and I'm sure it probably put her in debt for the rest of the year.'

The day I was given a red BMX bicycle I was made up, chiefly because it meant a faster getaway from the busies and what I felt was constant disapproval back home. There's a family photo of me with the bike in my prized (hand-me-down) Man United strip, looking dead chuffed. I quickly lost interest in cycling, though, and went back to my first love of football while keeping as far away from the house as I possibly could.

Thirty-something years later and halfway across

Canada, I was 5,400 miles away from Manchester and on a far superior bike to that first BMX as I took on my Dementia Adventure. Incredibly, Eric and my mum had stayed together until her death, and I'd learned to accept him. I think it helped that their early fears for my future had been allayed by my long and happy career in the Army, which had undoubtedly been the making of me.

By the time I was preparing to leave the military, my mother was sixty-six, and her anxieties about her sons were quite different than those from our rebellious teenage years – and far darker. Her eldest boy Anthony was virtually helpless and on the verge of going into an old people's home, and it looked like I was headed for much the same destiny. I can only imagine the unhappy memories seeing Tony must have brought back for her about Dad's final years in the Parkside Mental Hospital.

At least with my crazy bike ride in the planning I was able to give her something positive to look forward to and focus on for a change. She worked at the checkout at Tesco's in Altrincham, where she'd told everyone she came into contact with how proud she was of her soldier son. Bless her.

Determined to live up to that pride, I wasn't ready to roll over just yet. I still had a few million turns of the pedals in me even though it kept pissing down. In a strange kind of way the rain made me feel more at home. With a town called Graham up ahead, the Canadians must have known I was coming – what hospitality! Then there was the aptly named Yellow Brick Road and the Winnie the Pooh monument to tick off my growing bucket list a few hundred miles further on. In my immediate future, at least, there was nothing but good things to look forward to.

If in doubt – smile.

3

'Do not follow where the path may lead. Go instead where there is no path and leave a trail. Only those who will risk going too far can possibly find out how far one can go.'

T.S. ELIOT

Dementia Adventure Diary, 23 May 2015, Manitoba Highway of Heroes, Canada

'Moose on the Loose' wasn't another eclectic song from my playlist but one of those Canadian road signs flashing past that you don't see every day. This one was near a town called Sunshine that completely failed to live up to its name in the grey drizzle. Once again, I was logged into 'www.Iamsoaked.com'.

I hadn't spotted any moose yet – loose or other-wise – but I had seen five black bears within the first few days, a sight that literally took my breath away. Most tourists enjoy watching wild bears from the safety of their vehicles, but when you're on a pushbike it's an entirely different perspective and I had to be extremely careful. Unless I came upon a wild animal too fast as I rounded a corner (as happened once or twice), I'd stop, let them see me and wait for them to lumber off into the woods. Some of the adult bears were bigger than a man and could have done me real harm. Fortunately their chief goal in life was food. As could be said of me, they're often described as 'a nose with a stomach attached', so they were far more interested in roadside garbage bins or human food thrown from cars to mither with a skinny little snack like me.

Other unusual road signs I spotted along the sweeping Canadian highways alerted me to 'Watch for Wildlife', or 'Deer Crossing'. I was told I was in a 'Bison Area' or warned of 'High Impact Zones' with silhouettes of stags leaping onto vehicles. Fire hazards seemed to be a big problem in the forests too, but there wasn't much chance of that in the weather I was experiencing. Even the lakes were still frozen.

Most of the time, I couldn't see much at all as my eyes were smarting from the bitterly cold wind, which was brutal in Ontario – a huge province whose motto is 'Yours to Discover'. What I discovered is that its hills are extremely deceptive – so many ups and downs, with shockingly punishing inclines. But then, hey, that's life. I was also constantly hunkered down, pedalling into the headwinds. There were few opportunities to 'buddy cycle', and I soon understood why I was the sole cyclist riding east to west. I might have travelled ten miles in a headwind but someone going the other way with the wind behind them would have covered twenty over the same period. This was the only direction I could feasibly have gone, however, otherwise I'd have had to cross

Alaska and Canada in the winter, which would have been suicidal.

I'd always try to stop and say hello to my fellow knights of the road when I could, if only to enquire about the terrain and the weather up ahead. The cycling community is very open and most were eager to offer advice and a friendly word, or to share complaints about the toll the roads were taking on us all.

After three weeks in the saddle I had some serious causes for complaint. I was cold, wet and hungry, my bum was numb, and my right knee was causing me some serious jip. I didn't appreciate it yet, but the bike I'd bought was a little too big for me and I wasn't sitting in the optimal position. One day, a few weeks in, I posted a sitrep: 'Frustrating day with delays, crazy truck drivers, no room at the inn, comms playing up – but covered over 110km!' With such conditions, I faced quite a lot of hardship in those first few weeks and there were days when Vicks persuaded me to stop because of the cold and my pain. But they turned out to be the least of my problems.

In all the planning she and I had done, we hadn't factored in that many of the stores and campsites I'd expected to take advantage of en route would still be closed for the winter by the time I arrived. This meant finding alternative sites to bed down, or spending far more than we'd budgeted for on motel rooms that often weren't worth the money, especially as I was only crashing for a few hours before setting off again at dawn.

Plus, I couldn't cook in a motel so I had to buy my meals. With all the energy I was burning on the highways each day, my normally voracious appetite was off the scale. I must have been consuming around 10,000 calories a day, and I'd munched my way through far more of my Army rations than I'd intended. Vicky's careful calculations on how much I needed to eat were designed so that I wouldn't lose too much weight. Fat chance.

My daily diet started with three bowls of porridge, heated up when I could with water on my Jetboil portable stove fuelled by gas canisters. Then I had sandwiches during the day if I could source some. If not then I'd slap some ham and mayonnaise into six baguettes and pack them for the journey. I hoped to reach somewhere each night where I could buy myself a high-calorie cooked supper of pasta or pizza. I particularly came to like the Timmy Horton's chain, where I'd devour a plate of their steak sandwiches. I also ate a lot of foot-long sarnies courtesy of the Subway chain and should have earned loyalty points at Domino's Pizza. Whenever I grew hungry again (which was frequently), I'd snack on nuts, chocolate and sticky protein bars, but I could never get enough food inside me and genuinely feared I might run out.

Water was another issue. As well as six one-litre bottles in my panniers, I carried a CamelBak two-litre pack, which is like a day sack in a plastic sleeve that strapped to my back and had a straw from which I could suck water on the move. I filled it up each time I stopped and added sterilising tablets to it every day to try to ensure I didn't pick up any bacterial infections. The trouble was, the pack soon got sand and grit in it – plus I drank so much that I had to buy additional bottles of mineral water, which were never cheap. That's if I could even find a shop that was open to buy them from.

At one point in the middle of nowhere in 'Friendly Manitoba', almost a month to the day after I left the UK, I posted a video online to show the long empty road stretching far into the distance. Then I pretended to be asking directions to the nearest shop. 'It's what? Two hundred miles that way? Or two hundred miles that way? Eh??'

Major Ian Booth, my first ever staff sergeant in the Army, commented: 'You were never good at map reading.'

That's a bit harsh, sir. I'm geographically challenged, that's all.

With no campsites where I could pitch my tent and many of the motels and trading posts closed too, I often had no choice but to sleep rough wherever I could. My childhood escapades in Bollin Woods served me well. What they didn't prepare me for were the bugs. I kid you not – the North American continent has every type of insect you can imagine. Vast annoying clouds of them. Each time I slowed down or stopped, the little buggers would pick up my scent – although to be fair my cycling clothes did hum a bit!

The bugs would then descend in a swarm to buzz infuriatingly around my eyes, mouth and nose before gorging themselves on my blood. There were biting midges they call 'No See 'Ems' because they're so small, and mosquitoes with the persistence of a hungry Gurkha. Then there were deer flies, huge carpenter ants, hornets, pine beetles and ticks. The worst by far were the black flies, which I soon came to develop a phobia about, but more on them later.

I've served in some bug-infested places in my life and in the jungles of Sierra Leone I caught malaria, but Canada really tested my limits. It was like nothing I'd ever known, certainly not from my childhood. The worst creatures we had buzzing around us in Bowdon Vale were lazy fat bluebottles, and they didn't want to feed on me day and night. There were also some irritating sand flies on the beaches of Wales, which was the only place I'd ever been to outside of Manchester until I was sixteen years old.

We never had holidays when I was little, but after my dad died we went to Criccieth in Cardigan Bay with Mum's friend Joan, her husband Bill and their twin boys, who were eight years older than me. We camped in tents, and Anthony and I ran wild and pinched food from the supplies – we always wanted more than we were given. Joan said that back then I was a 'mischievous Jack-the-lad with a glint in the eye'. She was one of many who often told me how much I looked like my father, with the same cheeky expression and olive skin, as if we were 'slightly foreign'. It's nice to know I inherited something exotic from him, and not just what we in our family refer to as the 'daft gene'.

We returned to Wales a few times with Joan, and also with my mum's friend Val Goulding and her family. It's only when speaking to these two women that I'm able to build up a picture of what my father was like and how happy he and Mum had been before the disease took hold. Val called Mum 'Dot' and the two women had grown up in the same street in Wythenshawe so she knew how tough my mother had it. Mum had been the youngest of three, one of whom died of a heart condition, leaving her and her sister May.

My mother was in her early twenties when she met my dad on a night out in Altrincham and they were both instantly smitten. Once they started courting they'd meet under the clock tower on Station Forecourt but Dad was always late. One day my mother arrived early as usual and waited in the library opposite to see him turn up in a fluster thirty minutes late and then pace around wondering where on earth she could be. When she eventually emerged, he cried, 'Where you been? I've been waiting here for ages.'

'No, you haven't, John Graham!' she replied. 'I've been watching you from across the road.' They'd laugh and then get on with their date. She can't have held his lack of punctuality against him, though, because not long afterwards, they were married at Altrincham registry office.

'John was a lovely guy and they were ideally suited,' said Val, who attended their wedding. 'He really was the love of her life and they made such a nice couple.' My dad was also the youngest of three children, and he worked as a fitter at the Budenberg Gauge Company in Broadheath, which made pressure gauges. After they married, he and Mum moved to Vine Cottages nearby, known locally as 'The Backs' because the properties were reached via a ginnel down the back of the Chinese chip shop.

'John was a very nice man, what we'd call a hail

fellow well met,' said Joan Hill, who lived next door but one. 'A gentle soul and a hardworking man, he loved his family, although he spent far too much time running around after his rather domineering mother for Dot's liking. None of us had much money so we'd visit each other's houses and natter while our kids all played. For a treat we might go to the pub or the Hale Cinema to see a film.'

Joan remembers how dementia first revealed itself in my father in his mid-thirties. 'We went on a family holiday to Wales and John promised to feed our cats but when we came home, all the doors had been left open and the house unlocked. Other days, he'd forget when his shifts were so he'd get up on a Sunday morning and cycle to the factory only to discover that it was closed. His memory got worse and everybody began to notice – especially at work.'

Like me, Dad spent a lot of time making light of his forgetfulness at first. He'd get our names muddled up and then pretend it was a joke, but when the disease tightened its grip on his brain Joan said it began to change him. 'Nobody really knew what was wrong but it was obvious it was getting bad, even though he was still laughing in the face of death. Then he started to get the shakes and developed mood swings. He was sometimes aggressive or angry, and would smash things in frustration. His own mother Hilda refused to accept that what he had could be hereditary – almost as if there was some shame in that or it reflected badly on her. In her opinion, if John was unwell then it must have been down to Dot. Nobody wanted to talk about it, or what it might mean for the children.'

Joan said that when Dad finally 'lost it', my mother found it impossible to cope. 'He'd drink anything and everything he found lying around – even bleach. She called one doctor and then another and eventually he had to go into hospital. There was a struggle and it was pretty horrible and very upsetting.'

I know. I was there. Sadly, that's one thing I do remember.

Once my father was a full-time inmate of Parkside, Mum used to visit him every week and was often driven there by Joan's husband. 'It was a proper asylum and it used to frighten her walking the corridors and seeing all those mad people. She hardly had any money and yet John still smoked about fifty cigarettes a day and would get very angry if she didn't take him in fresh supplies. She tried to get the staff to stop him smoking – she didn't see the point – but they said they wouldn't intervene; it wasn't something they could easily do and would be against his human rights.'

I have no recollection of my father smoking when I was a kid, but then I have so few anyway. I do recall that Mum smoked and how much I hated it. She gave up for a while but took it up again later. I could never stand the smell, or the way it clung to my clothes after I'd been in her company. Perhaps because of that, I never smoked a cigarette or took a drug in my life. It just wasn't my thing.

Joan said that Dad escaped from Parkside a couple of times, often making his way to the local pub for a pint and a smoke. Then he was moved to a secure ward. 'They didn't put him in a straightjacket or give him electric shock treatment or anything like that. They just sat him in a chair where he chain-smoked constantly and slowly deteriorated. He was partly sedated so as not to mither anyone. He didn't even recognise Dot in the end.'

My mother, meanwhile, fell apart. She had at least one nervous breakdown after he died and left her with four kids and no money. For a time she was hospitalised, although she did eventually rally and found that keeping busy helped her cope. 'She had a lot going on and this is her story as much as anyone's,' Joan added sadly. 'I became her social worker, to the detriment of my own family. I even contacted the NSPCC and went to social services at one point, but they said they couldn't do anything. I was worried what would happen to the children. In the end I couldn't help her any more.'

Each time I think of what Mum must have gone through, I can't help but feel sorry for her – and for my dad. Out in the wilds of Canada with no one to talk to apart from Vicky and with music playing in my ears, I had plenty of time to consider what had happened to them both and what Vicky and I had yet to face. Most of the time I was a bit of an ostrich and tried not to think about such depressing things. I wouldn't say I don't worry about it – the thought definitely affects me – but I joke about it in a squaddie kind of way, which distracts me and helps neutralise the fear. What I do know is that the only certainty in life is death. I am not a martyr by any means, but I am being forced to consider dying at an earlier age than most.

Am I scared? I don't know. I've never died before.

With those kinds of thoughts spinning round my head, I quickly came to appreciate that this trip was going to be as much of a psychological challenge for me as a physical one. This was the first time in years – and certainly since my diagnosis – that I'd been entirely on my own, and although that gave me too much time to think, I was surprised by how much I was enjoying my own company and actually preferred being alone.

It was also incredibly humbling to be one insignificant bloke alone in the middle of nowhere sleeping under vast galaxies and shooting stars, or beneath a huge pale moon. Being something of a daydreamer, I'd gazed at the sky all my life, but in remote places where there wasn't any light pollution from a nearby town or city, it became a whole different scene. Even by day, most of the skies I saw in the land famous for being 'Big Sky Country' were utterly astonishing. I'd stop my bike sometimes just to watch an unusual cluster of clouds forming, and I always loved to see the sun come up – marvelling at the way it slowly tinted the earth different hues.

'I'm the only human being right here right now watching this,' I'd tell Shirley prosaically, 'and this sight will never be exactly the same again.'

Out there on my own I could cut my own detail, to coin a military term, and remain with my thoughts. For hours on end as I followed the natural contours of the land I could disappear into the geography of my own mind. Those who know about these things would probably say I was practising some form of meditation as I allowed my thoughts to drift constantly between the present and the past. I don't know about that, but as a long distance and marathon runner, I'd always enjoyed the solitary nature of the sport, with only the pounding of my running shoes against the ground to focus on. This time my rhythm was dictated by the revolution of my pedals.

Left, right, left, right...

The people I waved at as I sped past their lives probably regarded me as a healthy young man in his prime, enjoying a cycling holiday. Little did they know what I was really up against. Whenever I stopped to chat with anyone at a store or campsite they were extremely friendly – especially once they learned that I was on a charity ride and had been in the armed forces, which has a massive impact in a country where patriotism isn't treated with suspicion.

Something I couldn't help but admire along the way were all the national flags fluttering proudly in the wind outside virtually every home and business – especially, once I got to the US, the Stars and Stripes. I was struck time and again by how proud the people of North America are of their own country, which was so refreshing to see. I'm as patriotic as the next man and happily hoisted a tiny Union flag on the back of Shirley, but if I flew a full-size one outside my home I'd probably be thought of as a racist, which couldn't be further from the truth.

I was also impressed by how darned appreciative Canadians and Americans are of their military, police, fire service and medics. Entire highways and bridges are named in memory of dead servicemen and women and, as a lifelong soldier proud to have been a member of Her Majesty's armed forces, it was an honour to stop and read about each of them and give them my personal salute.

Calling up Vicks at one such site, I held up my camera phone to show her a huge plaque to fallen Canadian forces personnel. 'How great is that?' I said. 'I can think of a few people who deserve a street named after them.'

'Me too,' Vicky said, laughing. 'You, for starters!' She asked how I was doing and assured me that I only had thirty more miles or so to go that day. 'I've called up the next campsite and they're open, they have Wi-Fi, and they're expecting you. Plus, I've looked at Google Street View and it looks like there's a McDonald's en route and a shop nearby so you can stock up.'

'Brilliant,' I told her. 'I'll knock myself up a brew when I get there and then I'll FaceTime you.'

'Don't forget to take your multivitamins,' she reminded me, anxious that I continue to swallow the omega oil capsules and vitamin E and B complexes that she'd read protect the cell membranes in order to keep me in optimal mental health.

'Yes, Ma'am!' I mocked before signing off with a salute. Switching over to music, I pressed shuffle and the song 'Something I Need' by Ben Haenow filled my brain. As with many of my choices, the lyrics seemed especially apt: *In this world full of people, there's one loving me.*

Perfect.

If in doubt – sing along.

4

'Life is like a ten-speed bicycle. Most of us have gears we never use.'

CHARLES SCHULTZ

Dementia Adventure Diary, 3 June 2015, British Army Training Unit Suffield (BATUS), Alberta, Canada

It had always been my intention to drop in on a few of my old military mates if I could along the way, but until I finally made it to BATUS after cycling two hundred and twenty-five miles in two days along the Trans-Canada Highway, I hadn't appreciated just how much I was looking forward to it.

Not only would I have the chance to rest my aching muscles for a few days, but I'd be able to sleep in a proper bed, shower as often as I liked, eat some hot food, and catch up on some essential bike maintenance. Expecting a bit of sympathy, I posted online, 'Hopefully it will also give my buttocks some respite.'

Vicky immediately quipped: 'Bone idle!! All you do is sit on your butt all day.' She, meanwhile, was preparing to go back to full-time employment to bring in some much-needed cash in between struggling with single parenthood and keeping me on target. Her role in my whole adventure had grown massively from how we'd first imagined it, when she thought she'd get a check-in call from me once a week. Instead, it became apparent early on that I couldn't be left unassisted.

Quite apart from the fact that so many of the campsites were closed until May, the mapping systems we used were designed chiefly for vehicles, not bikes, and didn't allow for the fact that cycling on interstate highways is against the law. Each day Vicky had to re-plan my routes to navigate me onto some of the older highways flanking the interstate. I had to rely on her more and more, to the point that she never felt able to go to bed until I'd finally stopped for the night, which was usually around three or four in the morning Zulu – GMT. Then, she'd be up early for Dexter and to get her daughter Katy off to school. I don't know how she kept going day after day, and I had no idea how she was going to manage work as well.

Incredibly, she kept her cool throughout and only lost it with me a couple of times – usually when we had no comms or my satellite tracker stopped tracking. One day I went missing for nine hours somewhere in the depths of Saskatchewan with no signals until I reached a motel, where the pings suddenly restarted but were very erratic. Vicky immediately thought, 'Oh, shit. Has someone jumped on him? Has he gone off the road or is he in a scuffle?' Her imagination ran wild as she couldn't think what was creating my unusual pattern of signals.

'I rang the motel but they said there was no one there by that name, which panicked me even more. Then the pings stopped altogether and Chris vanished off the face of the earth. I was pacing the floor and on the verge of calling the mounted police when he finally contacted me at five thirty a.m. The first thing I said was, "Where the hell are you?" He confirmed the name of the motel I'd already called and then when I rang again, this time a different receptionist said, "Yes, Ma'am," and put me straight through to his room. I almost died!'

We discovered later that the reason for my odd ping pattern was that I'd accidentally put the Yellowbrick on the wrong setting. Vicky patiently talked me through pressing the right buttons to return it to the normal setting and was finally able to calm down. As she often told people, 'I had a few sleepless nights but it wasn't me out there with dementia, pushing against the clock and dodging bears. I never forgot that what Chris was doing was phenomenal.'

With hindsight, we probably should have done the whole thing differently and organised care for Katy back home. Then we could have hired an RV – a recreational vehicle, or motorhome to you and me – and had Vicky follow me each day and help me set up camp each night. I wouldn't have needed to haul the trailer, I would have saved a fortune in food and accommodation, and I'd have had the added bonus of seeing her and Dexter every day.

Thanks to her invaluable assistance from afar, though, I was actually starting to feel a bit smug as my journey was going so well. I'd been averaging a hundred miles a day instead of my intended forty and I genuinely wondered if I'd be away as long as I'd originally thought. 'Will it take a year?' I mused online. 'Who knows? At the moment I feel fine. I am sure something will slow me down. So it's good to be a little ahead of time.'

My route thus far had taken me through mile after mile of the same kind of country – predominantly pine trees and lakes – in the region of western Ontario and Saskatchewan known as 'The Land of the Living Skies'. The ride from a place called Bruce Mines on the north shore of Lake Huron to Sault Sainte Marie, close to the US border, had been surprisingly good, with an unexpected burst of warm weather that brought out the butterflies, enhanced the scent of pine sap and kick-started dazzling displays of wildflowers. The welcome sunshine also started off my T-shirt and cycle shorts tan nicely (I'd look like a Newcastle United fan by the time I was done).

Once I got to Sault Sainte Marie (pronounced Sioux Saint Marie), though, the heavens opened and everything was soaked again. The whole place seemed very run down, and was full of 'First Nation' Ojibwe people from the settlements – Native Americans to you and me. I was surprised by the hostility and racism I encountered towards them, as they seemed to be generally regarded as no good or on the piss. I have always made a point of saying hello to anyone I meet, whatever their class, creed or the colour of their skin – I'd chat to the devil, me – but I could tell these people were not only extremely poor but dead wary of a white face.

There were few facilities at the campsite I stopped at in town and nobody was about, so I began to think tactically. I was fed up with getting wet each time I stopped to put up my tent, as it meant I'd either have to wait for everything to dry out or put it back on wet before setting off again. I recce'd the location like the squaddie that I was and looked around to suss out where I could put my head down with the least hassle. That night I ended up sleeping on the floor of the one-person lavatory block, rolling out my sleeping bag right next to the toilet pan. I've slept in worse places in my life, but not many.

Lights out!

That was also the night I opened the first of Vicky's three envelopes, which I'd kept in my driest pannier to protect them from the rain. Tearing at the paper, I pulled out a printed card decorated with colourful hearts which read: *Whenever you are feeling sad and things aren't going right, and your usual happy smile has slipped out of sight, here's a little hug from me if I cannot be there because I want you to know just how much I care.*

Feeling better already, I left the remaining two envelopes sealed – just in case – although I never opened the others until I got home.

In spite of her cheery message, those first few weeks continued to be my toughest thanks to the general lack of facilities, the brutally early starts, the unexpectedly rough terrain and the frequent changes of weather. Quite early on, dogs started to be an issue for me too – strays mostly, but also pets who were so territorial that when I cycled past

71

their owners' property they came after me, sometimes in twos or threes, to snap at my heels. Fortunately, I had years of experience with sergeant majors and adopted a strident tone to yell at them, which usually stopped them momentarily. Failing that, I'd use my air horn. The trouble was, I wasn't on a racing bike. It was more of an oil tanker and I couldn't get away fast enough. I was lucky that none of them bit me.

Pushing on towards Thunder Bay I navigated some punishing hills. Then my front disc brakes needed attention, which made for interesting cycling – especially downhill. Fortunately, Vicks found me a bike shop online and they sorted me for the next leg, which was just as well. I was soon head down in wind, rain and Force 10 gales, whilst continually dodging juggernauts. Move fast and stay low, the Army had taught me, and that was precisely what I was doing.

The weather did let up long enough for me to tip my hat to the Winnie the Pooh statue in White River, one of several monuments to celebrate the black bear cub bought from a trapper by Canadian Lieutenant Harry Colebourn in 1914 and transported to London as a regimental mascot. The officer left young 'Winnipeg' or 'Winnie' at London Zoo while he served in France. Among the thousands who visited the zoo to see her was Christopher Robin, the son of writer A.A. Milne, who admired her so much that he renamed his teddy bear after her. The rest, as they say, is history.

Crossing time zones, it had been far from dry in Dryden (oh, the irony) and the beautifully named

Lake of the Woods proved to be a picturesque mosquito breeding ground. In the midst of a deluge and with extremely sore muscles, I rode through the sprawling city of Winnipeg and on to some brilliantly named places such as Moose Jaw, French River Trading Post, Jack Fish, Loon, Wild Goose, Swift Current, Antelope and Medicine Hat. The largely deserted roads were dotted with signs warning 'Caution Wildlife on Highway', so I remained vigilant for bears all the while.

Wildlife wasn't my only concern. One day as I was cycling through the wilds of Ontario on a two-lane highway with forests left and right, something dead strange happened. The roads were so quiet that I'd only seen three cars all day. Pausing for a moment, my feet firmly planted either side of the crossbar to make sure Shirley and my trailer didn't topple over, I stopped for a pee, a snack and a drink – in that order. Ever since I'd wet the bed as a boy, I seemed to need to use the loo more than most – I often quipped that I had the weakest bladder in NATO. Now that I was drinking several litres of water a day, I found myself in almost constant need of relieving myself and there was rarely time to get off the bike and find somewhere private.

Using SAS-style initiative, I worked out how to do what I called a 'stealth pee', which involved me doing what I had to do straddled either side of my bike, whilst pretending to look at a map and hidden by a small bag I had strapped to the front of the bike. It worked every time.

Once I'd done the business, I turned on the satnav, checked my position and then dialled up

Vicks so that she could help me plot the rest of my course for the day. There's a saying in the Army – if in doubt, ask. The more my memory was failing me, the more I knew I needed to check and double-check everything and keep second-guessing myself. A mistake out there on the road could be fatal.

I had my earphones on and was listening to Vicks chatter away when I suddenly heard the sound of an approaching vehicle. Looking up, I saw a dark green pick-up truck coming slowly towards me. I was even more surprised when it stopped immediately opposite where I was resting up.

'That's odd,' I said quietly to Vicky. 'Someone's here.'

'Who?' she asked, sensing the change of tone in my voice. 'Who is it, Chris? Are you okay?'

I didn't respond but watched out the corner of my eye as a big fat guy aged about forty-five with straggly black hair and a beard got out of his pick-up and stood staring at me. The hairs immediately rose on the back of my neck. I'm a marathon runner but standing in the position I was in, I couldn't have moved anywhere very fast. I'd have been better off away from the bike, but I couldn't risk leaving that either, so I carried on munching on my sarnie and tried to stay calm.

'Hey man, can you help me with something?' the stranger called across the highway. I felt strangely comforted that Vicks could hear every word. Not that she could do anything, mind.

'You what, mate?' I responded in my best Manclish.

'I need your help,' the man said, still staring at

74

me as if I was his next meal. 'I need to get something out of the back of my truck.'

I tried desperately hard not to look as frightened as I felt. 'What?' I said, bristling.

I heard Vicks cry, 'Get out of there, Chris! Don't go near him!'

I lowered my sandwich and shouted, 'Why the fuck would you stop here in the back of beyond to get me to come over to your truck?'

He didn't speak and just kept staring. I prayed he didn't pull a gun on me.

'Chris? Chris?' Vicky's mounting panic was evident.

Pretending to be wryly amused and trying to defuse the tension, I asked him, 'What have you got in there anyway – an alligator?'

'No, man,' he replied, his face deadpan. 'I just want you to get something out of the back.'

Angry then, and even more annoyed that he was frightening Vicky too, I told him firmly, 'No, I'm not fucking helping you. Why have you stopped here? Do you think I'm stupid or something?'

He shrugged. 'Gee, I only wanted your help.'

'Well forget it. Now get lost.' Using a well-known Manchester insult, I cried, 'Just do one, will yer? You dick!'

I could have cycled away then, but I chose to stand my ground and stare him out as he stood cursing me. In the ensuing silence, Vicky listened, holding her breath. Very deliberately, I said something to her to let him know that I was connected to the outside world. Then I finished eating the rest of my snack and calmly set off, keeping a close eye on his movements in my wing mirrors. I say 'calmly' but I honestly thought my heart was going to leap out of my chest.

There was no question in my mind that he was a bad man who wanted to entice me over to his vehicle for some reason. If anything terrible happened to me out there nobody would have known except for Vicky, who'd have heard it all unfold on the telephone. Her biggest nightmare up until that point had been that I might go missing on this trip and that she wouldn't know what had happened to me. She feared that because of my condition I could get confused, take a wrong turn, lose my way and end up dying of dehydration or a broken leg in the wilderness. Her only comfort was the fact that the Yellow-brick had a red emergency button I could press that would send an immediate alarm signal to the company, giving my exact coordinates and letting people know I was in the brown sticky stuff.

Neither of us had factored in the prospect of me being murdered.

If the sinister stranger had chosen to turn and come after me, I'd have been in real doo-doo. Had he shot at me or tried to run me down, I'd almost certainly be toast. I updated Vicky on my progress every few minutes as I sped away, continuing to watch him in the mirrors until he was a tiny black dot in the distance. Even so, I kept an eye out for him for the next twenty miles or so, afraid that he might still come after me. I only wished that my old army muckers were a whole lot closer than they were, so it came as a huge relief when I spotted the first signs to the camp.

Although I'd served in North America a few

76

times, I'd never been to BATUS – the British Army's largest training facility in the world for armoured and tank exercises, live training and Arctic warfare. It also has a large British Forces Post Office (BFPO) through which all mail to our forces serving in North America passes, so I was keen to see if any of my former shipmates were there.

Having finally accepted that a serial killer wasn't hard on my heels, I raced across Alberta as fast as I could. A few miles into what is known as 'Wild Rose Country' I hadn't spotted a single wild rose, but not far from Suffield I hooked up with an old mate called Mark Precious who I'd known since my earliest days in the Army. He'd left the services and married a Canadian, and he lived in a town called Maple Creek where I enjoyed some quality R&R. Then, once I neared BATUS, I stopped and shacked up at the house of Stan Hogg, one of my first sergeant majors and another top bloke.

When I arrived, he was planting trees around the lake in his garden and decided to plant one in my honour – or so he said. Maybe he just wanted me to do the digging? Either way, he told me, 'We'll give it a name and then each time you come and visit you can watch it grow. So, what's it to be?'

'Easy,' I replied with a grin. 'Gurkha.'

Although I didn't sleep in the barracks but in one of Stan's nice comfy beds, I did spend a lot of time in the camp saying hello to old friends and making some new ones. I had my photo taken with some of the lads outside the BFPO, where I'd hoped to pick up some mail from Vicky, including

77

an all-important new SIM card to keep my phone costs down. Sadly, it hadn't arrived. The good news was that I was able to ditch some of my kit. The GoPro camera had been a mint idea but I wasn't very proficient and hardly ever used it, taking snapshots on my phone instead, so I handed it over, plus a spare satnav and a few other bits and bobs, to send home to Vicks.

I didn't know that many people at BATUS as there were a lot of Canadians there, but everyone I met was kind and gave me every encouragement. I had hoped to stay at a lot more army camps along my route as, in the good old days, any veteran with a military ID could spend a night there for free. But due to higher security the rules had changed and the practice had been stopped, which sadly prevented me from hanging out with a few like-minded lads. The camaraderie of Army life was definitely what I missed the most from my days in uniform and, in many ways, it also re-minded me of my four years in children's homes as a kid.

I'll never know what it was that finally tipped my mother over the edge the year after Eric moved in with us. Whatever it was, she was prompted to call in social services and ask them to take Tony and me away. I know he'd been misbehaving and I'm sure I was a little swine by then, driving Mum up the wall. My sisters were angels by comparison and only ever got into trouble whenever we led them astray.

Tony and I had been grounded almost every night for a year, but he blatantly ignored his cur-few and I continued to climb down the drainpipe and onto the ledge before jumping down and heading off to the river or the woods. With my dark skin and wild ways I earned the nickname 'Jai', after the native boy in the TV series *Tarzan*, which all the kids loved. Even when I go into the local pub now as an adult, someone will often cry, 'Hello, Jai!'

I was certainly rebellious and sneaky, dodging chores whenever I could. In fact, if Mum asked me to do something, I'd leg it. She'd chase me as far as York Street and then give up. I must have been near impossible to discipline but, in my defence, I wasn't a truant and I did still go to school every day – if only for the sports.

Tony was sent away first. In 1986, when he was fourteen years old, he just vanished from our lives and no one dared ask why. He started off in a children's home but was then fostered by a middle-aged couple from Manchester who were devout Christians. After a while, we lost all contact. Val Goulding said that my mother couldn't read or write that well and didn't realise that Tony would be taken away for good. 'She said later that she was given something to sign but didn't know what it was and only discovered later that the move was permanent. She was very upset and thought the system had let her down.'

Tony remembered it slightly differently and said Mum had appeared in person at the court hearing where his fate was decided. Whatever the truth, she lost him then – we all did – and her once-adored firstborn Anthony never returned home.

I don't even remember being particularly

shocked that my big brother was gone. He'd been leading his own life for so long that I didn't really miss him at first. Tony had always gone his own way, a fact that intrigued me and only made me long to be his mate. I was much closer to my sisters, especially 'Busy Lizzie' who went to the same school as me.

What did shock me was that I was taken away soon afterwards. I was twelve years old and nobody warned me. Our soon-to-be-condemned council house might have been inferior, but it was the only home I'd ever known until Mum and Eric decided they'd had enough of my lawlessness. Two male social workers arrived one day and marched me out the front door as my mother stood silently by. My saddest childhood memory is of sitting in the back of their van feeling very scared as it was driven away down our little road. I'd hardly ever left our neighbourhood before. It was all I knew. I wondered where they were taking me and what it would be like. Would I be bullied – or worse? Would Tony be there? When could I come back home?

My destination turned out to be a children's home called Beechmount in Langham Road, Bowdon, just a mile from my house. It's a smart apartment block now, with asking prices we'd never have believed in a million years, but back in 1988 it was a place for kids who'd broken the law. Once registered and searched, I was put into a dormitory with loads of other lads and abandoned. Looking around me nervously, I had no choice but to get on with it.

Stand by your beds!

Although it was frightening at first, being there wasn't nearly as bad as I'd imagined it to be. In many ways it was better than being at home. The building was warm, dry and clean and I was served hot food every day. The kids weren't the best types to be associating with, but many were there through no fault of their own, including one lad whose mother had been murdered by Peter Sutcliffe, the Yorkshire Ripper. I was the youngest and the smallest of them all at less than five feet tall, but I never got picked on, probably because I was cheeky enough to get away with most things. Even when I grew to the dizzy height of five foot seven in adulthood, I always claimed it as an advantage, jokingly announcing that I was too small a target for enemy fire.

I made friends at Beechmount quite quickly but within two weeks I was moved away to a much bigger children's home in Sale, on the other side of Altrincham. It was called Northenden Road, and it had two wings housing thirty boys and girls. Once again I was very apprehensive at first, but it was okay and for the two years I was there I was allowed to travel to my old school and back every day, which made me feel less isolated and allowed me to see Lizzie every day at break time. I wasn't ever really angry with my mum for sending me away; I think I mostly felt sorry for her. I was more pissed off to be so far away from all my mates, as I had to go straight back to the home after school each day and couldn't play football or mess about by the river like a pirate any more.

Mum didn't sign any permanent removal papers for me and, to be fair, she did visit once or twice to ask me if I wanted to go home. I told her I didn't. I never liked Eric and although he'd steadied the ship, so to speak, I blamed him for me being in a home in the first place. After a while, she stopped asking and then she stopped visiting.

Whenever I got too homesick, I'd run away for a few days just to spend time with my friends and to see Lizzie. The police would come looking for me, but I'd hide on the allotments or hang out at a friend's house watching Arnold Schwarzenegger videos. His unsuspecting parents had no idea I was 'missing'. One time I camped out for a couple of nights in the shed of a house opposite ours, where Lizzie sneaked in to see me every day, bringing me sandwiches and fizzy drinks. She'd have done anything to spend time with me and hear more of my stories. At eleven years old, she missed me dreadfully, especially when Angie grew old enough to be out on her own with her friends, leaving Lizzie home alone. Mum and Eric had a year-old baby by then, our half-sister Alison, and when the council decided to do up our entire terrace they were all moved to a housing association property ten miles away in Oldfield Brow.

When Lizzie saw how well fed I was in the children's home, she started to feel jealous. She was so envious of my trendy new shell suit that I immediately gave it to her, knowing they'd buy me a new one. 'I kept asking Mum if I could be sent to the children's home too,' Lizzie said later. 'Chris seemed so happy there and was having a good time.'

What I never told her about were the nights I

was desperately sad because I missed everyone so much. I didn't say how much I resented all the restrictions we had to live under, or how I hated not being able to play football or get into mischief with Neil Deadman, Craig Calder and the rest of my mates. Like Neil, Craig lived on Bollin Avenue around the corner from me. He was such a happy-go-lucky kid and he quickly became one of the lads. I definitely didn't like being in the children's home all the time, especially when I was going through puberty and all the emotions that go with it. But I needed some strong role models and the mostly male staff members there were good to me and never cruel, so I was lucky.

One day, not long after I'd arrived at Northenden Road, I received a phone call, which was a first for me. Hard as it is to imagine these days, I'd never used a telephone in my life and I didn't know what to do. I picked up the receiver gingerly and held it to my ear as a voice down the line said, 'Hello? Is that you, Chris?'

'Hello?' I replied, half afraid to speak into the device that reminded me of a walkie-talkie I'd seen in war films. I almost added, 'Over.'

'It's Tony,' the disembodied voice said.

'Who?'

'Anthony, you idiot. Your brother.'

'Oh ... hi.'

'Someone told me you'd been put in that place so I'm calling to see if you're all right.'

'Oh... Okay.'

'Well, are you? All right, I mean.'

'Y-yes. I'm okay.'

'Good.'

There was a long pause. Then he said, 'So I'll call again if you like. You know, just to check on you...'

'Yes ... great.'

'All right. Well, bye then.'

'Bye...'

I held the receiver in my hand long after he'd gone. I hadn't thought to ask if I could call him – not that I'd even know how. True to his word, Tony did call me again, every month or so, just to check up on me. That's when I first realised with a warm feeling inside that he did want to be my mate after all.

He was still living in Manchester at that time, working at Gateway supermarket in Stretford Mall, so I asked Lizzie one day in the school lunch break if she'd like to go with me to see him. She'd forgotten what her big brother looked like, but she never forgot that day. 'We went to Gateway and waited round the back for Tony to finish his shift. I remember standing watching those plastic flappy double doors they have into cold stores and was so excited that Tony was going to walk through them. He seemed pleased to see us and we walked and walked for miles just talking and then he took us back to his flat. It was great.'

Not long afterwards, I pinched a bike for Tony so that he could get around more easily and maybe even come to visit me. I thought he'd be pleased that we could be mates but he knew it was nicked and, now that he was a Christian thanks to his foster parents, he told me off. Soon afterwards, he just disappeared. It was a while before I found out that he'd moved to Newtown in Powys with his new family. He was eighteen when he met his future wife Janette at a local church youth group there. He gave up his rebellious teenage ways and took a job in a supermarket in their small market town. Bizarrely, when Mum and Eric went on a camping holiday to Wales and she nipped in to buy something, she came face to face with Tony at the checkout.

Val Goulding said, 'Dorothy bumped into Anthony by accident somewhere quite remote. She had no idea he was there but was very pleased to be back in touch with him.' It took Tony a long time to forgive Mum for sending him away, and he never invited her to his wedding to Jan in 1995, but I think he did forgive her in his own way – eventually.

Aside from Neil and a few old friends from primary school, nobody else knew I wasn't still living at home. It was another part of my life I chose not to share. One of my oldest friends is Rachel Curwen – we were in the same tutor group at Wellington Road Secondary School for five years – and from the outset we got on like a house on fire. Rachel was one of the few people who knew I was the only kid at our school living in a children's home, but she never let on.

'It wasn't widely known,' she admitted later. 'It only came up because we were chatting one day about where we lived. He never said why he'd been sent there and I never asked. I just accepted it, in the same way that I accepted he had quite a trek each day to get to school and could never come home for tea or to play at the weekends or in the holidays. He had such a tough childhood but he never complained and was always so inspirational to me.'

Quite rightly, Rachel claims that I was always a handsome devil with loads of thick hair, which I wore as a flick across my eyes. One Direction, eat your heart out! She added, 'Chris was what I'd call a loveable rogue. He struggled a bit at school and was a bit absent-minded and not one for retaining information, but he brushed everything off with a laugh. He was always chirpy and full of beans, as if things bounced right off him. He didn't have very much money and could never afford Christmas or birthday presents, but I always got him something. Quite early on he decided that as soon as he left the children's home he was going to join the Army. I never doubted it.'

Carry on, soldier!

After two years at Northenden Road, I was moved to Marple Grove children's home in Stretford, which was even further away. From there, I had a long bus ride to school twice a day. The first good thing that happened, though, was that I was signed up for a local football team – the Unicorns. Derek Hale, the coach, took such a shine to me that he volunteered to pick me up after school and drop me back to the home after games, or I'd never have been allowed to play. That cheered me up no end, especially as Neil was in the team as well. So he and I were able to reconnect.

The next good thing was that, having been kicked out of the cubs for getting into a fight during a football match, I was accepted into the Army Cadets in Sale. Finally, in cadet school I found the order and discipline I'd secretly been craving. At last, I got to put on the khaki uniform I'd longed to wear ever since the Falklands War. I soaked up everything they taught me like a sponge, learning how to square bash and practising my drill. I studied the weapons systems and memorised the various ranks. I took unaccustomed care over polishing my boots and looking after my kit. I competed in cross-country running competitions and we visited several army camps to get a flavour of the life. I loved being in the military, from the day I joined as a snotty-nosed teenager to the day I left as a grown man.

For almost three decades, I wore my uniform with enormous pride, and the recent loss of it and my Army career was still very raw to me. Being around soldiers again at BATUS in Canada was really great but it also became something of a bittersweet experience, reminding me of all that I was missing. After a few good days spent in the company of some great lads who hosted me with fantastic generosity, I was ready to get back on the road and continue my adventure on my own.

If in doubt – soldier on.

5

'When the spirits are low, when the day appears dark ... when hope hardly seems worth having, just mount a bicycle and go out for a spin down the road, without thought on anything but the ride you are taking.'

SIR ARTHUR CONAN DOYLE

Dementia Adventure Diary, 13 June 2015, Trans-Canada Highway, Alberta, Canada

Having seen little but trees for weeks, I found myself in the dead flat prairie lands of central Canada. As far as my eyes could see there were vast fields of corn and then even more fields, dotted every now and again with farms or towering grain stores.

This was a landscape that offered no shelter or respite from whatever Mother Nature decided to throw at me. And she hurled some pretty extreme weather at me for the first few days after I left BATUS, so much so that at one point Vicky made me stop again.

'You're pushing yourself too hard, Chris,' she chided. 'Unless you rest now you'll be going nowhere tomorrow.' It grew quite tense between us at times as I always argued that I wanted to crack on, but she was usually right and forced me to acknowledge how tired I was. I've always been good at obeying orders, so I did as I was told and pulled in at the next campsite. Posting online, I wrote: 'Due to very strong headwinds and heavy rain, I've decided to take an enforced admin day and wait for the weather window to pass. I was riding against it all day yesterday. Sometimes the juice isn't worth the squeeze!'

Speaking of squeeze, I'd developed a painful medical problem that Vicks and I had never factored in. Over the previous few days, I'd been feeling more numb than usual down below. I'd given up wearing underpants early on because the seams rubbed against my skin with each rotation of my legs, so I went commando under my cycling shorts (well, I was entitled to, after all!). The trouble was that about three weeks into the ride, whenever I stopped to have a pee, nothing happened – just a drip, drip, drip. The longer it went on and the more I drank to rehydrate, the more it hurt, until I was in agony.

'This is killing me, Vicks,' I texted her. 'I think something might be seriously wrong.'

'Let me look it up,' she texted back, and within a few minutes she was on the phone, reading to me from a website that explained in graphic terms what was happening and why. 'It's prostatitis,' she said. 'Also known as Cyclists' Syndrome. The pudendal nerve in your prostate is being squashed or entrapped by being in your saddle all day. It says here that, untreated, this can cause erectile dysfunction, inflammation in the penis and pain after sex...'

'Stop right there!' I cried, panicking. 'Tell me what I have to do!'

'You need to get to a bike shop and change your saddle, pronto, soldier.'

She texted me the address of the nearest bike shop, which was about thirty miles west, and I rode there as fast as I could, hobbling in like an old man.

'Yup, we see this kind of thing all the time,' the cheerful salesman told me, completely unfazed. 'You need a saddle with a hole in it for your kind of endurance cycling.'

'Do you have one?' I asked, almost cross-legged.

'We do,' he replied, pulling a rather strange-looking saddle out of a box. Taking one look at the pained expression on my face, he added: 'Once we've fitted this, my advice to you is to go find yourself a bath and have a long, hot soak. Then try using the bathroom. That should do the trick.'

Mercifully, he was right and the problem squared itself away at a nearby motel. I don't think I have ever felt such intense relief in my life.

At ease, soldier.

With my bits hanging free and easy over the specially grooved saddle with its elongated hole, I was back on the road again in no time. This time it felt like I was floating on a cushion of air. I had to laugh out loud when one of the first songs that shuffled onto my playlist was 'Swings Both Ways' by Robbie Williams. Yes, siree!

With the skyscrapers of Calgary behind me, I hit the nursery slopes leading to the mighty Rocky Mountains that loomed ahead of me, covered in snow. A brake failure soon had me limping into a town called Red Deer for some parts, but I maintained my sense of humour and after that I was on my way again, eager to get to the peaks.

Of all the sights on my journey, I think that those mountains thrusting themselves skywards from the earth were the first that truly impressed me. I stopped to take some photos but I could never really do them justice; they were just too fantastic and made me feel so grateful to be alive. The clarity of the air and the beauty of everything up there on what felt like the top of the world gave me an enormous rush. It was so humbling. After a few more hours of sensory overwhelm, though, it became a bit ridiculous as I found myself stopping at every new corner to be staggered – yet again. At this rate, I'd never get anywhere.

Near Calgary I turned north towards Edmonton on my way to the Yukon, the province known as 'The Land of the Midnight Sun'. I'd be cycling the east flank of the majestic Rockies and eventually crossing them further up at a place called Eureka Roadhouse, 'Gateway to Alaska', at 3,300 feet above sea level. My ultimate destination for this particular leg was at a distance of 2,050 miles and a few weeks away in Anchorage, in the American state known fittingly as 'The Last Frontier'.

In mid-June, I posted a sitrep video from a remote spot about four hundred miles outside Edmonton. 'Good morning all, as we speak now I'm en route to Fort St John, which is about ninety miles away. The weather's not too bad although you can see in the background that the clouds are forming already. Today I go into British Columbia and another time zone, so hopefully the weather will hold off and I'll speak to you soon. Ciao!'

When I boasted the following day about how

easy this cycling lark was, Vicky was quick to remind me that I'd be meeting up with her and Dexter in Vancouver soon, something we'd planned from the start to keep my spirits up and so she could check on me. 'Ha ha,' she commented. 'Make the most of it. Your five-month-old clone is going to be keeping you very busy in five weeks' time!'

I couldn't bloody wait.

Throughout my long cycle round, I received loads of other encouraging comments from friends and family that always gave me such a boost. My sisters were amazingly supportive and my mate Neil Deadman wrote, 'Keep going brother. All so proud of you and following every mile you cover. Keep the updates coming and the not-so-hilarious videos!! You're a hero to many and I'm proud and privileged to know you! Now get a f$%*!g move on!!!'

That made me laugh and I told him, 'Bro, I want to get back for the start of the footy season.' Which was true. I hadn't seen a Man United game in months. Once a Red…

At my next rest stop I did a load of washing in the sink to get the sweat and salt stains out of my clothing. Whether I put my things back on wet or dry didn't really matter, because if they were dry they'd soon be soaked with sweat and if wet and it was hot, they'd dry out in minutes. I posted a photo of my tent and my washing hanging on a line draped across a picnic table. 'A cyclist's job is never done,' I wrote. 'Can you believe I have to do my own washing! Shocking, do they not know who I am?'

Vicks joked, 'I sincerely hope you aren't saving the next load for when I get there next month!!' And my former classmate Rachel added, 'About time. We could smell you from here.'

There was nothing for it on these long stretches between major destinations but to knuckle down and keep my wheels spinning. I had a few hard days in the saddle with some nasty headwinds. I encountered sticky heat and torrential rain, plus the bugs, which were a constant niggle. Sometimes the rains were so bad that I literally stripped off and packed my clothes away so they didn't get wet. Then hailstones the size of pebbles would blow in to pummel me. Some were so big that I watched them strip trees of their leaves. There was rarely any shelter from lightning as I waited half-naked by my (metal!) bike praying I didn't get struck, but then I figured that I'd probably already had my share of bad luck already.

The winds continually bothered me because I could easily get blown off my bike, as had happened once or twice. That was extremely dangerous when I was clipped in. I already had quite a few bruises on my hip and some grazes on my legs. The wind also blew bugs and grit into my eyes, which felt like little stones at speed. So I started wearing sunglasses, and eventually I was given some ballistic goggles.

Vicks kept an eye on the weather forecast each day, as well as the wind speed and direction, looking ahead of my route to assess what I might be headed into. She was really thrown in at the deep end, having to learn all this stuff.

'You're probably only going to manage about

fifty miles today,' she'd warn. 'There's a steep incline and the wind will be against you.'

One day she made me stop halfway through a mint ride on what seemed to me to be a perfect day. 'There's a supercell storm system brewing. In about forty miles you're going to run straight into it. There's a whole lot of nothing coming up with no shelter or campsites. You're going to have to stop there.'

Although I knew that if the weather turned I needed to be prepared, I was quite grumpy about it that day because the sky looked clear as far as I could see and I didn't want to lose time. She was the boss, though, so– 'Yes, dear.' And she was right, of course. She was the brains of the outfit and I was just the monkey on the bike. Thanks to her forward planning, I can honestly say there were only one or two moments when I genuinely felt like I'd had enough – and they were mostly down to the wind or the bugs, which she could do nothing about. Mostly, I felt surprisingly calm, listening to music that triggered memories of different countries and different times in my life, while communing with nature.

Because I didn't make any noise I was able to see much more wildlife than anyone in a vehicle would have done. I spotted moose, more black bears, deer and other animals long before they saw me and usually by the time they did, I'd whizzed past. I was grateful again then for my wing mirrors, so that I could see what was coming up behind me too. The last thing I wanted was a grizzly on my tail. I'd read somewhere that they could run as fast as 35 mph if they put their minds to it, and I had no intention of becoming meals on wheels.

I was a lot more aware of the wildlife when I was wild camping, and extremely wary of them coming hunting for food. That's why I always followed the tried and tested advice of hanging food or anything that gave off a scent high up in a pannier, suspended on a rope slung over a branch several feet away from my tent. The worry was that I'm such a sound sleeper I wouldn't have heard anything until a predator was upon me. I was completely alone at one campsite when I woke up in the morning to find the large industrial bin nearby completely upturned and trashed. Only bears could have thrown that bin around – big bears at that – but I hadn't heard a thing.

Another time, I rounded a corner and came face to face with a herd of bison either side of my two-lane highway. Larger than cows and with Viking-style horns, these snorting hairy beasts were grazing on a nine-foot strip of grass on either side. I was right in amongst them before I knew it. I did think about stopping and waiting for them to move on but they looked like they were perfectly happy to stay put. I didn't want to spook them, so I slowed right down to about one mile an hour as they all looked up. Quietly, I unclipped my feet from the pedals so that I'd be able to do a runner if I fell off, and carried on moving very slowly through them, looking right and left all the time. There were several calves and I tried not to get between them and their mothers, but they were all so close I could smell them and even feel the warmth of their grassy breath.

Increasing my pace a little, I was alarmed to see that some of them began to speed up with me. I went a little bit faster and they started running alongside me. By the time I'd crept up to about five miles per hour they were quite literally galloping along with me, their hooves pounding the earth and throwing up great clouds of dust. It was all rather surreal, as if they thought I was one of them somehow. They ran with me for about a hundred yards before they finally gave up. Looking back at them with relief, I knew that the whole encounter could have gone horribly wrong, but in a strange way it was also rather magical.

I had another close encounter of a different kind one morning after wild camping in some extremely remote spot. As usual I woke early to brew some tea and get on my way. As I sat outside my tent in the dawn light, a chipmunk approached me without any fear whatsoever and sat back on its haunches to stare at me. I'd spotted a few raccoons and I think I saw a skunk on the road once, but I'd never been up close and personal before with one of these native squirrels in what looked like a Sunderland strip.

Maybe I'd been on my own too long, but I really felt like he and I made some sort of connection in those few moments. We were locked onto each other with direct eye contact. I didn't say a word but I couldn't help but wonder what the little fella was thinking as he sat, whiskers twitching, staring at me. While I was musing on his innermost thoughts, the bugger darted forward, snatched one of my precious Earl Grey teabags and ran off! I had to laugh, although I probably should have skewered the little tea leaf and eaten him for breakfast.

I've never met a soldier who doesn't love a cup of tea and I definitely developed a taste for it in the military, where a brew, or a 'wet', was almost always on offer. I was soon hooked. Not that the staff manning the Army Careers Office in Fountain Street, Manchester, welcomed me with a cuppa to begin with, mind you. When I first turned up there in 1991 aged fifteen and a half and looking much younger, they regarded me with some bemusement, handed me some leaflets and told me to come back once I was old enough. In spite of expressing my absolute clarity that this was what I wanted to do, I had to wait until my sixteenth birthday and go with my link worker from the children's home, who carried proof that I was of legal age to sign up.

In my schoolboy heart I secretly wanted to join the Marines or the Paras as a commando. Ever since the Falklands War and the successes of our rapid reaction forces there had sparked my interest in the military, I'd been determined to get the green lid – the beret that can only be worn by a British commando. I'd also read a lot of books about the various elite corps of the military whilst I was in the cadets. Beggars can't be choosers, however, and my time was running out. I was about to leave secondary school and would be moved from Marple Grove children's home into a sort of halfway house for kids like me. I didn't want to do that, and I had no intention of going back to live with Eric and my mum.

I was told that if I signed up to something called

the Junior Leaders, the youth training regiment for the British Army, I could join virtually straight away. Because the system was changing, though, I could only become a member of the Royal Engineers. Otherwise, I'd have to wait six months. I didn't want to wait another day. 'What about doing a commando course?' I asked.

'There'll be plenty of chances to try for that kind of thing later, sonny,' I was told. It didn't look like I had much choice in the matter, so I went to see my mum to get her permission to become a boy soldier.

'If this is what you really want,' she replied. I think she was relieved that I had a plan and wasn't going to drift into aimlessness after school. With her blessing, the relevant papers were signed and I had a full medical and sight examination before completing all the necessary tests. As always with exams, I found the academic side of things much harder than the physical, but I concentrated hard and somehow managed to scrape through. Once I'd passed, I dragged my mate Neil down there to try to get him interested in signing up with me, but we both knew Army life wasn't for him. I was on my own.

Before long I'd been given a date to report to barracks – 29 June 1992. My mother tearfully waved me off from Manchester Piccadilly station and I remember thinking rather coldly that it was strange that she should cry when I hadn't even lived with her for years. Nothing, however, could dampen my excitement that I was getting on a train to Chepstow in the Welsh borders to start my Army career.

Looking around the rail carriage after I'd changed at Birmingham New Street, I spotted several other teenage lads with kit bags and quickly introduced myself. Some of the friends I made that day have remained mates ever since. As usual, I was probably the smallest amongst them and I was also the only one who didn't have any stubble, being such a late developer. In fact, when they taught us how to wash and shave during our first week I had nothing to take off, to be fair, as I'd only recently sprouted pubes!

I quickly fell in with the military life, and didn't even mind relinquishing my famous lick of hair for a short back and sides. One of the first things I learned was all about the call signs the Army uses to identify each member of a troop and every location without giving anything away to an enemy. So I might be call sign HO1 (Hotel Oscar One), speaking to HQ (Zero) and giving my log stat (location) as M23 (Manchester) on my way to London (L21). Once everyone had that learned, then it became common to refer to each other merely by their unique call signs or simply just as 'callsign'.

One thing that was new to this callsign was being ordered to attend church every Sunday. I'd rarely been inside one and I'd much rather have been out running or playing footy, although I did enjoy the singing. As I sang along at the top of my voice, I wondered if that was what my born again Christian brother Tony most liked about church too.

For the next ten months, I was just one of a gang of lads who'd been thrown together to be treated like shit by our commanding officers. It felt a bit like being in prison. The friendships I made there served me well for the rest of my life and when the film *The Shawshank Redemption* was released and I watched it with my fellow soldiers, I realised that not only were there parallels with Army life but that I was probably the least homesick of them all. I'd lived away from home for years, I already knew how to make my bed, keep my locker tidy for daily inspection and look after my kit. I'd learned all that the hard way. To this day, I could watch that movie over and over and never tire of the hero Andy Dufresne surviving the unthinkable and finding a brilliant way to escape from the horrors of his life.

There were other things I had to learn the hard way, too. On one exercise in the Brecon Beacons, a lad I was running with hurt his back and couldn't carry his 30lb Bergen another step, so I offered to carry it for him. 'Thanks, mate!' he said with genuine gratitude as he struggled on up the hill behind me. Happy to take on the challenge, I made it to the top where I threw his kit down and sat on it to catch my breath with my own Bergen still on my back. Our sergeant was waiting to bark at us.

'Sapper Graham, whose kit is that and why the hell are you carrying it?'

'One of the lads is injured, sir,' I responded.

'Well, well, aren't you the little Johnny Gurkha?' he sneered. 'You even look like one, especially as you're a bit yellow and such a short arse.'

The name soon stuck and I've been known as 'Gurkha' or 'Gurkhs' to my army mates ever since.

Being likened to one of the fearless Nepalese soldiers known as 'The Bravest of the Brave' was no bad thing, I figured. It was certainly preferable to 'the midget', which is what a few of them called me.

I learned so much at Chepstow and sailed through my basic training. Mum, Angie and Lizzie came with Eric and Alison to watch my passing-out parade and I knew then that I'd made them all proud in my crisp uniform and shiny boots. My next move was to Gibraltar Barracks in Aldershot in Surrey for Phase Two and my six-month B3 combat engineering course. There I learned how to defuse mines, tie knots, use tools, make concrete, construct and demolish bridges, fill sandbags, manage water supplies, dig holes and become a general handyman. We were loaned out to create an adventure playground from scratch and had to cut steps into a sloping bank for some country pursuit enthusiasts.

Once again, I struggled with the academic modules, especially the dreaded theory papers in which I had to memorise a load of facts and figures, but I got by. Whether it was an early indication of my dementia or whether I just wasn't the sharpest tool in the box, we'll never know, but I've got the best excuse in the world – blame it on my genes. What I loved most were the physical fitness tests, including a four-mile run (piece of cake) and a five-mile loaded 'tab' or march (easy peasy) plus a military swim test. I was grateful that I'd taken myself off to Altrincham Baths as a nipper and taught myself to swim.

Apart from all the physical challenges and

learning about basic engineering, I was also given a taste of the different trades in the military to see which appealed to me the most. It was this module that changed my life forever.

If anyone had told me when I first signed up to the Army that I'd become a 'postie', I'd have laughed in their faces. But my time working alongside members of the Royal Engineers Postal and Courier Service (now renamed the 29 Postal Courier and Movement Regiment) was a real eye-opener. The service is one of the British Army's oldest units, dating back to the days when King Edward IV organised a courier network of armed horsemen between London and his armies in Scotland to deliver vital orders and dispatches. Since those earliest days, trained soldiers have been accepting, sorting and delivering mail to facilitate military planning around the world for the Army, Navy and Air Force. We set up secure field post offices and more permanent BFPOs and then received and carried official as well as personal mail to the front lines, in order to maintain order, keep lines of communication open and raise morale.

Formed as an official military unit in 1882, the service is now part of the Royal Logistics Corps but originally came under the remit of the Royal Engineers' Telegraphers because the maintenance of roads and telegraphs was such an important factor in keeping lines of communication open. Even with the invention of email, a postal courier service is still vital to guarantee secure delivery of orders and mail in remote areas without the internet.

I didn't know any of this to begin with, of course. And I certainly had no idea I'd be sent out with just my rifle and a couple of equally nervous colleagues to open up what were often considered to be unsafe routes in places like Afghanistan, Bosnia and Kosovo. All I knew at seventeen was that because every unit and each military exercise require the services of the posties, they don't remain stuck in one place with their unit waiting to be deployed like regular soldiers, but travel in much smaller groups all over the world. With only a couple of trips to Wales under my belt, I was itching to see more. I never once regretted my choice to join the proud regiment whose motto is simply 'We Sustain'.

Having completed my training at the Postal and Courier Depot in Mill Hill, north-west London, in 1994, I was posted to Dalton Barracks in Abingdon, near Oxford, where I was to be officially based for five years. With my first proper soldier's wages, I bought my mum a spin dryer and a few extra little things to make her life more comfortable. It was the least I could do.

Ian Booth was my staffy – staff sergeant – in Abingdon and became a lifelong friend and ally. He was older than me and taller than me (most people are), so I had no choice but to look up to him. He was handsome, fit and – as I frequently joked – 'hung like a well-endowed field mouse'. I owe him a lot. It was from Abingdon that I truly began my world travels with one plum tour after the other, each of which presented me with new learning opportunities. Over the next five years these included two six-month tours of Bosnia as part of the UN force, as well as training exercises in Turkey and America, to mention just a few. I was part of the Allied Command Europe Mobile Force (AMF), a small NATO multinational force that could be quickly dispatched to demonstrate the solidarity of the alliance and its ability to resist aggression against any member state. To relax away from the stresses of the job, I developed my love of running and the older I got, the better I was at it. Well, I'd always managed to outrun my mum, so I reckoned I was virtually born match fit.

In May 1996 I was invited to take part in Exercise Purple Star in Fort Bragg in North Carolina – the biggest combined US-British deployment since the first Gulf War, involving more than six thousand troops including Paras and Commandos. When it was finally over, my sergeant told me almost casually, '45 Commando need someone from our detachment to go with them to Twentynine Palms in California for an exercise. They've got a man down. Do you want to go?'

'I can't believe you're asking, sir,' I replied. 'Train with the commandos?'

Yes, sir!

It was my dream job to spend time with the elite of the elite for three months. I learned a great deal about endurance fitness once I joined their daily PT sessions. Yes, I was in good shape and had always been a competent runner, but I realised I didn't have the kind of core strength I'd need to become a commando, so on my next tour of Bosnia I developed my own schedule and trained like ten men – running, rope climbing, press-ups, sit-ups and pull-ups.

When we were given time off in the US a lot of the lads elected to drive to Las Vegas to go gambling and see some of the shows. I chose instead to join a few of the other commandos and climb Mount Whitney, the highest mountain on the US mainland, which towers over Sequoia National Park and part of Yosemite. It's a steady walk rather than a climb, but at 14,500 feet a lot of people had problems with the altitude, although I was fine. Standing on the summit with a bunch of elite soldiers was one of the high points of my life, if you'll excuse the pun.

It was my experiences in California that made me decide to try to fulfil my childhood dream, so I applied to undertake the commando course myself. Ian Booth had recently completed it and he spurred me on. In his words, 'Chris wanted that badge so badly, he wouldn't take no for an answer.' With running as my chief form of exercise, I'd go for a ten-mile run with some mates and then come home and set off immediately on another, and then another.

'Chris is the fittest bloke we've ever met,' some of those friends told Vicky the first time they ever met her. I'm not sure whether they were trying to impress her on my behalf or scare her off, but she already had an inkling that I was physically robust.

It paid off in the end because by the time I got to the Commando Training Centre in Lympstone, Devon for the first two-week 'beat up' to see if I'd be up to the full endurance course, I was in the best shape I'd ever been. I was all set to start when disaster struck. Out in a pub in Altrincham with

105

my mates on the Saturday night before I went back down to Lympstone, I slipped coming down a spiral staircase and badly sprained my ankle. Within a few minutes, the joint was swollen and bruised and I could hardly put any weight on it.

Gutted, on the Monday I limped in to see the Royal Marine captain (who looked like Desperate Dan) and told him what had happened. Judging from the expression on his face, it was touch and go whether I'd be kicked off, as the course was already over-subscribed. Luckily for me, when he called up Boothy to tell him he was pulling me out, my staffy told him, 'No, let him crack on. He's a good lad and he's trained hard for this. Give him a chance.'

Dosed up on painkillers and with my boot laced up tight to support my ankle, I managed to get through the next few days, which fortunately were at a slower pace. We were on the rifle ranges and the parade ground learning field craft skills. Then, as the pressure mounted and we were faced with tests of physical strength, flexibility and endurance, my tender ankle seemed to hold up well enough for me to get away with it. Mercifully, it was squared away by the time we got to the assault courses, battle swimming tests, climbing, rope work, speed marches, and massive night-time runs in full fighting order over the rugged Dartmoor terrain. More than a hundred of us started that course but less than thirty finished, and most failed themselves. Even Superman would have found it tough.

After nine gruelling weeks on the moors, I passed every test first time. Not only did I complete the final thirty-miler in full kit with a 31lb Bergen but I was presented with a certificate of commendation for being one of the best on the course. Boothy handed me a bottle of champagne when I'd finished. I was over the moon. I'd finally earned the right to wear a green beret at any training establishment and could sport the tell-tale red dagger on my left sleeve to prove it.

Becoming a commando was definitely my proudest moment and something I'd wanted to achieve since I was a little boy. Although I was confident that I could manage it, until the day I actually received my badge of honour I didn't know if I really would, and that was such a top feeling.

Whatever else had happened in my life – what I'd already gone through and was yet to face – I was officially a good soldier, which was all I'd ever hoped for. After commando training, my Dementia Adventure would surely be a piece of cake. If I could complete both before the curtain fell on my life then I would know that I'd done all right. Who knows? I might even have made my late father proud.

If in doubt – Gurkha on.

6

'Life is like riding a bicycle: you don't fall off unless you stop pedalling.'

CLAUDE PEPPER

Dementia Adventure Diary, 24 June 2015, Liard River Hot Springs Provincial Park, British Columbia, Canada

There isn't much that gets me down. I'm lucky that I don't seem to have the kind of personality that lets life beat me. I guess I inherited the sunny side of my nature from my father, so that's another thing to be grateful for.

But even my poor old dad would have lost his famous sense of humour if he'd had to encounter the shocking hordes of flesh-eating black flies that dogged me as I edged my way across Canada. I'm not at all surprised that they're known as a scourge to livestock and have been known to kill cattle, horses and even the occasional moose. The poor animals die from shock, toxaemia or blood loss. I only hoped the bugs sucking my daft blood would get dementia from it.

Needless to say, I found it utterly soul-destroying having to dodge them all the time, and pitching my tent at night was often the worst part of my day. If a campsite had a water source nearby, especially if it was standing water, then I knew immediately that there would be a problem. I'd jump in the water and wash off the sweat that seemed to attract the buggers, but almost as soon as I got out I'd have to don my full mosquito suit with netting hat and gloves, an outfit that I even had to wear cycling in the most heavily infested areas. Still they came for me.

On the day I put a photo of myself online in my full mozzie kit, several of my mates enjoyed a laugh at my expense and joked it looked like a 'gimp suit'. A former PT instructor of mine commented, 'Somehow that's arousing me.' Another military mate said, 'I thought for a second you were wearing a burka.'

Then in the middle of Canada, somewhere not far from the Rockies, the black flies defeated me. When a cloud of them locked onto my stink and descended, I was more frightened than I'd ever been in my life and simply couldn't go any further. They scared me more than the bears. In my wing mirrors I could see the swarm coming after me and I did my best to outrun them. At times I performed a kamikaze manoeuvre by riding dangerously close to trucks or huge RVs in the hope that the flies would be blown back in the slipstream. It would take at least ten attempts to blast them far enough away, but still they persisted.

Desperate, cycling for my life, I called up Vicks and cried, 'Babes! Find me a motel! I've got to get under cover!'

'What? What time is it there?' she replied blearily.

'Midday I think,' I cried, swatting flies as I pedalled furiously. 'I can't stand these bloody flies a minute longer!'

She called me back a few minutes later with the name of a motel four miles away and I rode like the devil to get there. The swarm was still in my wake as I quite literally dumped Shirley on the ground, ran to the front door and banged on it, yelling 'Let me in! Let me in!' I didn't step one foot outside until it was dark and I knew that it was only the mosquitoes I'd have to contend with.

When Vicky told me that she'd booked my next rest day at a place called Liard Hot Springs I thought at first she must have lost her mind. 'Hang on, won't there be loads of flies at a place like that?' I asked.

Good girl that she was, she'd thought of that. 'The water's too hot for them, apparently,' she replied. 'It'll be great for your sore muscles though.' She was right. Slipping into that open bath in the middle of a beautiful spruce forest was so relaxing. The slightly sulphuric-smelling water was around 50 degrees Celsius and, although I was embarrassed by my random tan, I soon forgot about that as I allowed my aches and pains to melt away.

Only after I'd settled happily round the campfire with a few fellow travellers did I discover that, a few years earlier and at the very same campsite, a man and a woman had been mauled to death by a black bear that also injured two others who tried to save them. Later that night, I was woken from a deep slumber by the loud roaring of male bears fighting in the woods uncomfortably close by.

'Shit!' I cried, sitting bolt upright in my sleeping bag and wondering what I might use to fend off a grizzly. I didn't sleep much after that. Less than a month after I'd cycled on, parts of the surrounding park were closed to the public following reports of 'significant bear activity'. Those are three words a lone cyclist and camper never wants to hear.

With all its critters Canada was proving to be somewhat challenging, and there were other unforeseen problems too. Up until I reached the Yukon I'd been lucky that Shirley hadn't had any major mechanical failures. I only had to put up with a couple of punctures, failed brakes, or attend to the chain a few times. The chain never snapped, but it stretched due to the weight I was pulling and the punishing mileage I was putting her through. I carried a couple of spares plus links, so I could usually fix the problem myself and crack on.

But when I got about four miles outside a remote place called Coal River on the Alaska Highway in British Columbia, something far more serious went wrong and Shirley began to make a terrible clanking sound. I'd just smugly posted a photo at the Yukon province sign which featured the slogan 'Larger than Life' when my brake system failed. Instead of pushing on as I'd hoped, I had to limp into an RV park on the Alaska Highway near the Muddy River Indian Reserve. This place was what Canadians call 'an historical' roadhouse, with parking for trucks and the numerous RVs the size of buses that were becoming a new menace to me on the roads. It also had a field for campers. There was a diner too, but unfortunately no one who knew anything about bikes.

'Can you tell me where the nearest cycle shop

is?' I asked the waitress after ordering two full cooked breakfasts (I'd decided against bison steak after my close encounter with those noble beasts).

'That'd be in Whitehorse,' she replied, scribbling down my order.

'How far is that please?'

''bout seven hundred kilometres.'

'Bloody hell. That's further than London to Edinburgh!' She looked puzzled so I asked, 'Where can I catch a bus?'

'Oh, that's easy. Right outside.'

'Great! What time does it come?'

Her brow furrowed with concentration. 'Well, today's Wednesday, so ... the next one will be Saturday.'

With only two buses a week and a journey time of at least twenty-four hours there and back, I knew I'd lose far too much time and risk being late for Vicky in Vancouver, which was out of the question. Looking around at my fellow diners, I noted that they were mostly truck drivers or older couples travelling in heavily laden RVs, few of whom would have room for Shirley, my trailer and me.

When I'd finished stuffing my face, I wandered outside somewhat despondently to try to call Vicky but there wasn't a phone signal. I bought a phone card from the camp store, called her up and told her what had happened. 'Listen, Chris, we can shelve us meeting in Vancouver if this means a huge delay or it's going to make you push yourself too hard,' she gallantly offered.

'No way!' I told her. 'Not an option, soldier.'

We signed off and I was wondering what best to do when a huge two-tanker fuel truck swung into the car park. To my surprise, a woman climbed down from the driver's cab. In her forties with a mane of black hair, she looked like the kind of woman nobody would mess with.

'Excuse me, madam?' I asked, in my cheekiest Mancunian (which most North Americans mistook for Australian). 'Do you mind telling me where you're heading?'

She looked me up and down in my full Lycra before replying warily, 'Whitehorse.'

'Brill,' I said, grinning. 'It's the only place for miles with a bike shop and I've broken down. Do you think you could give me a lift?'

I could see her hesitation so I blurted, 'I promise you I'm not a murderer or a rapist and I'm happy to pay something towards your petrol.' I couldn't help but smile at the irony of that, given the load she was carrying.

I think she found my accent both difficult to understand and rather amusing, and she laughed out loud at my use of the word 'petrol' instead of gas. 'Okay,' she replied, shrugging.

'Cracking!' I cried before clapping my hands together and pointing to my rig. 'Now where can I put my bike?'

I'm sure at that point she instantly regretted offering me a lift, but between us we managed to haul Shirley and my trailer up onto the roof of her tanker and strap her down with elasticated bungee straps. I then gave her my panniers containing all my valuables to put in her cab. Not taking into account that Vicks had no idea what

113

I'd arranged for the journey to Whitehorse, I took a picture of Shirley on her side on top of the tanker and texted it to her without any explanation. Then we set off.

I've completely forgotten the lady's name but I'm going to call her Mindy. She ended up being incredibly helpful and not nearly as scary as she looked. I quickly discovered that she had some serious back-up on board, because when I climbed into her cab I came face to face with two slobbering Staffordshire terriers who travelled everywhere with her. With her devil dogs and her husband in Whitehorse on speed dial in case of emergencies, she had all angles covered.

Mindy was a top driver and drove like the professional that she was. A woman of few words, she pushed on through a land once only occupied by gold prospectors, fur trappers and traders. When night fell, she pulled into a truck stop for something to eat and to bed down in her cab. I unpacked my tent and set it up right next to her tanker. Early the next morning I woke up to a frantic message on the Yellowbrick from Vicky, who'd been up most of the night. Having received my cryptic text, she'd been following my fast-moving pings on the tracker and wondering what the hell was going on and why she hadn't heard from me in over two hundred and fifty miles. She was beside herself.

'Sorry, babe. I've had no phone signal and I've hitched a ride from a tanker driver,' I texted her back quickly. 'I'm all right and we stopped for the night. Don't worry, she's sound and she's married. I'll call you when I get to Whitehorse.' I could only imagine her thoughts as our conversation came to an abrupt end.

Even with several thousand litres of fuel on board, my Good Samaritan drove like there was no tomorrow and we finally reached Whitehorse later that day. Mindy kindly dropped me right outside the only bike shop in town and even brought her husband along to meet me later. They were both really good people.

The bike shop recognised my rig as a standard tourer and soon found the necessary parts to replace the brakes and deal with the latest effects of wear and tear. They admired my Kevlar-lined tyres but were less impressed when I told them that they weren't as impervious to punctures as I'd been led to believe. After an hour or so, they'd sorted me out and directed me to the bus stop, where I loaded Shirley into the cavernous hold of a Greyhound bus for a rest and travelled all the way back to the RV park. Once at the diner, I got another health-conscious meal inside me before setting off on the long road back to Whitehorse, following the same route I'd just traversed twice at speed.

Quick march!

This time my journey, punctuated only by mesmerising white lines or the swooping shadows of birds of prey, seemed to take forever. At night I ended up sleeping rough in places where I caught a whiff of the wild and had the eerie howl of wolves to serenade me to sleep. It made me wonder what it must have been like for the 100,000 or so 'stampeders' of the Gold Rush in the Klondike in the late 1800s, when thousands of people rushed to the Yukon to seek their fortune. I read somewhere that each of them was required to bring a year's supply of food to that untamed land in order to prevent starvation. I had every sympathy.

Out there I was back to the long silences of the wilderness, where all I could hear was my own hard breathing and the spinning of the wheels on the road. I had nothing but my shadow chasing me for mile after endless mile. Unless I found somewhere I could chat to Vicky for free, our snatched if frequent conversations were – by necessity – mostly focused on my day's ride so as not to use up too much of my credit or battery power. Even if I'd locked into someone's Wi-Fi, more often than not I'd contact her from the khazi during my evening constitutional. Well, it was warm, dry and quiet in there – and as I had the runs for the first four months thanks to the enormous quantities of food I was consuming, the toilet became one of my favourite places.

'Chris Graham, are you FaceTiming me from the loo again??' was her familiar complaint the minute she saw me stripped naked – the only way to peel off my figure-hugging Lycra onesie.

'That's classified, soldier,' I replied, smiling.

'Urgh. Call me back when you're done!'

I've always been a sociable bloke and it felt good to pull into a campsite or enter a diner and start a conversation with someone. Most people who saw me arrive would immediately be intrigued by my rig, which suggested to them that I was travelling a long way. Curious, they'd wander over to check it out and ask me where I was headed. 'I'm on a

116

charity bike ride around North America,' I'd tell them with a smile. Then, to get it out of the way, I'd add, 'I've got dementia. It's in my family and I'm trying to raise awareness and money for research.'

Almost everyone was instantly sympathetic. Nine out of ten would tell me they knew someone with dementia and share their own sad stories. More often than not, I'd be invited to their tent or RV for some food, which was always welcome. Often they'd try to give me money for the fund, but I'd direct them to my Just Giving website. 'That's really kind, thanks,' I'd tell them, 'but I don't take cash and I'd lose it anyway. I need to keep it transparent so that's the best way to donate.' One old boy in his nineties insisted that I accept the twenty-dollar bill he pressed into my hand. I'd only stopped by the side of the road briefly somewhere for a drink when he came out of his house and started talking to me. 'Take it, sonny,' he said, his eyes watery and his face lined with age. 'Buy yourself something to eat. You're going to need it!' It was always such a boost to meet folks like him and I can't thank them enough for their generosity of spirit.

One couple in an RV even kept pace with me for a time after I first encountered them at a campsite in Fort St John. Doug Mason was Canadian and his wife Jenny was British and they were travelling with their dog. Like many RV drivers, they were retired and had decided to drive around America in something the size of a small house, but for which they needed only a regular driving licence. Many of their fellow RV owners even towed a car on a fixed hitch behind, extending their length by several feet.

Jenny and Doug were the exception, but a lot of these elderly 'kings of the road' didn't have the skill or experience to manoeuvre their giant machines on narrow roads and were a menace to other road users, especially cyclists. The fact that they are almost entirely self-sufficient with food, fuel and water on board also inadvertently led to the closure of many of the more remote rest stops along the main tourist routes – places that may have appeared on a map but were long shut by the time I arrived.

As the Masons' planned route was going to almost mirror mine, we caught up with each other at various campsites and agreed to try to hook up again if the timings worked out. It was good to know there'd be a familiar face and a hot meal waiting.

The thing I liked most about being in the Army was the travelling, but the second best thing had been meeting so many fascinating people along the way, just as I was doing again on this trip. Many of my fellow soldiers had become lifelong friends and I was touched by how they continued to encourage and support me from afar. There are too many of them to mention, but one friend I've never lost touch with is Andy Harrison, known to one and all as 'H'.

He and I were in Chepstow together and he was all set to be a combat engineer until he broke both ankles pole-vaulting, so he joined the postal service and me. When asked what he most remembers about me from those early days, H says, 'Even at eighteen, Chris was known for being stupidly fit. We'd go out on runs with the physical training instructors and he'd always be up front and then he'd overtake the PTIs, which annoyed them so they'd speed up and we'd all have to follow suit. We'd be shouting, "Slow down, Gurkha!" as we fought to keep up. Anyone else would have pissed people off for that, but Chris was always so outgoing and friendly that we forgave him. I've never met a more genuine person.'

H and I served in Vitez and Sipovo in Bosnia together in 1990 as part of the UN peacekeeping force. The war was still going on so we never stepped outside without a weapon. We took a few incoming rounds on our convoy and were shot at randomly too. One day a couple of mortars landed about a hundred metres away and that certainly woke us up. In hairy moments like that, it's good to have someone watching your back.

One of our PTIs at Abingdon was Mark Swift, who was a corporal in the postal service when I started as a sapper. Swifty says of me, 'Chris always reminded me of a Jack Russell dog; he was so full of energy and enthusiasm. He had his nose in all sorts of things with a true terrier spirit. He stood out for being fit and was very keen to throw himself into everything.'

Pete Davies is another fantastic shipmate, who I first met in Abingdon in 1997 soon after I'd completed my commando course. He and I were both lance corporals in the postal service and hit it off straight away. 'Chris is infectious,' Pete said. 'He's such a positive guy and he's up for anything

119

and won't take no for an answer. He's lived his whole life that way.' From the day I told him about my diagnosis he was eager to do whatever he could and he's never let me down yet. While other people were patting me on the back and wishing me luck – never quite believing I'd manage the bike ride on my own – Pete was the one saying, 'There are no ifs and buts. Chris will do this. The only thing that'll stop him is if a bear eats him or someone shoots him, I reckon.'

Thanks, mate.

Then when I was posted to the Duke of Gloucester Barracks in South Cerney in Gloucestershire, I was one of three posties who became known as the 'dream team' or the 'three amigos', because we were sent to so many dodgy places together. The other two were Jason Marshall and Carl Cox. In 2001, after the New York Trade Center attacks, we were all sent on tour to Afghanistan for five months with 2 Para and 16 Air Assault Brigade as part of Operation Fingal. We were some of the first into Afghan, which was in a desperate state with security nowhere near as tight as it should have been.

The Taliban were being kicked out, but they were still resisting and frequently deployed suicide bombers. It was before any camps like Bastion had been set up, so everything we needed had to be flown in via air freight. We had no vehicles to start with, and when we did receive them they had limited fuel. We always had weapons – SA80 rifles and Glock or Browning pistols – but only so many rounds of ammunition each, and none of us were issued with helmets or body armour.

With very little infrastructure and no internet, our task was to establish postal routes secure enough for the delivery of top secret, diplomatic and other mail. Every day we had to drive thirty minutes through snow and ice to the airport to collect the mail and then drive the fifty miles from Kabul to Bagram along a road littered with ordnance. The risk of dying in a traffic accident or being blown up by an IED – an improvised explosive device – was our biggest danger, especially as we weren't in Warrior armoured personnel carriers, just a small convoy of regular Land Rovers. Several Allied soldiers were blown up in those early days and there were random attacks by gunmen, so there were genuine dangers to be faced every day. We had orders to set fire to the mail and especially to destroy any top secret documents if we were captured, or if it looked like we might lose them to the enemy.

Once our day's work was done we returned to our quarters in a semi-derelict office building we'd requisitioned on the outskirts of Kabul. They were extremely basic. There were no showers and it was so cold we had to chip through the ice each morning to shave. I hated sleeping twenty to a room so I set up my tent just outside the building, which suited me better despite the chill. It also proved to be a blessing when a series of severe earthquakes struck in early 2002, killing at least two thousand civilians, injuring twice that number and leaving thousands homeless. The quakes and the aftershocks even woke me up from one of my deep sleeps, making me jump out of my tent. I watched a streetlight swaying like a reed with the tremors and heard the alarmed cries of the lads inside the building, where the whole thing must have felt much worse and they feared the roof would cave in. Fortunately, none of them was injured.

One of the biggest daily hardships for me personally during my tour in Afghanistan was the fact that to begin with there wasn't a proper canteen. We had no choice but to subsist on half rations, which meant my stomach thought my throat had been cut. I used to dream about going to my local chippy for pie and mash, or fish and chips with peas and gravy, and wake up salivating. By contrast, my mate Pete Davies was based in five-star accommodation in Bahrain at the time, so he jumped on a plane to Bagram air base with a nine-kilo mailbag full of goodies such as coffee, chocolate and breakfast goods delivered to my tent. Now, that's what I call a diamond geezer.

No matter how bad the conditions, we 'three amigos' always had a laugh – often at the expense of others. Posties are notorious for pinching things for our various squadron bars – especially flags and signs from foreign tours. Known as a sticky fingers since childhood and encouraged by my captain, I once shimmied up a flagpole in Turkey and nicked a huge red Turkish flag for our collection.

My greatest coup by far, however, was pinching a large metal sign the size of a table from outside the headquarters of Airborne Logistics in Kabul. The moment I spotted the sign, which read, *Airborne Logistics: You'd Better Sort Yourself Out*, I knew we posties had to have it. Late one night, as we were on our way to Kabul airport, I jumped out of our Land Rover with a screwdriver, quickly unfastened it and threw it into the back. It was in the hands of the posties in Oman before dawn broke.

What I hadn't expected was the enormous fuss there'd be about the loss of this sign. Everyone blamed everyone else and senior officers went on the warpath. I'd have got away with it if the bloke in Oman had done as he was asked and mailed it back to South Cerney, but instead he kept it in his tent. With an amazing stroke of bad luck, it was spotted by the very officer who'd bought it for his unit in the first place. Reclaimed, it was finally returned to the regiment, a little battered but still intact. With even greater irony, I ended up being based in Nepal years later with that same officer and – during a long run together – he stopped suddenly while we were talking when he suddenly twigged I'd been the culprit all those years before. Of all the officers in the British Army, what were the odds of that? He couldn't help but be amused, though, and after grinning and calling me a wanker, he carried on running at my side.

I was lucky that I didn't get into more serious shit than I did over that, but in the end I think they saw the funny side. I was a fit lad in a green beret so, after ordering me to make a donation to a local charity, I was let off the hook. Happy days.

Practical jokes aside, Afghanistan was – without doubt – my most dangerous tour, only made bearable by the company of good friends. Every time 'You're the Voice' by John Farnham came around on my bike ride playlist I couldn't help but think back to those times and remember us singing, *How long can we look at each other down the barrel of gun?*

Feeding on those memories as I pushed on towards Alaska and the most westerly point of my journey, I was looking forward to reaching that major milestone. In my simple way, I imagined it would feel a bit like reaching Birmingham when you're on your way north to God's own country (Manchester) and you know you're almost there. From Anchorage, I would turn south to start my long journey down the west coast of America – hopefully, out of the headwinds that had been wearing me down since Ontario. Once I reached my halfway point close to the border with Mexico, I would turn again and head east. Months and months further down the line, in what sometimes seemed like an unachievable goal, I hoped to hook up with my mate Pete Davies who had promised to fly out to Washington DC and cycle with me for a few days.

But first I had another very important rendezvous to make, and one that was far closer to my heart. In the coming weeks, Vicky and Dexter would be flying out to Vancouver so that we could spend a precious twelve days together. For almost two glorious weeks my long-haired colonel would be with me in the flesh, not just a voice in my ear or a blurred face on my phone. I could hardly wait and they were just a hop, a skip and a cycle away.

If in doubt – pedal harder.

7

'Whenever you find yourself doubting
how far you can go,
just remember how far you have come.'

UNKNOWN

Dementia Adventure Diary, 12 July 2015, No Man's Land between the Canadian and US borders

I'm not sure when I first started talking to my bike Shirley, but I think it must have been quite early on. It wasn't long before I began talking to myself too, muttering away all the while as I fretted that I might have forgotten something important.

Each morning and every night I talked myself through a series of OCD rituals that involved painstakingly crosschecking my route and then my kit to ensure that I didn't mess up or leave anything behind. Once during my travels I left the Yellowbrick and had to get it mailed on to me, which did nothing to endear me to Vicky and began to make me paranoid. Even after I'd carefully gone through everything I'd worry that my mind was playing tricks on me, so I'd ask myself, 'Did I just do that?' There was so much to remember and I'd often lose my train of thought and tell myself, 'Focus, Gurkha.'

Attention!

Like everyone in the military, I'd been trained from an early age to check and double check my kit and never leave anything behind that could cost me my life or give the enemy an advantage. If I set off without one of my tent pegs or a piece of vital kit, then I almost certainly wouldn't realise until twelve hours later when I was setting up camp again a hundred miles further on. By then it would be too far to go back and I might well have to pay the consequences.

My panniers had to be checked and balanced each time too, and I always gave Shirley a thorough shake-up each morning to make sure that nothing untoward had happened to her overnight. If I came off in the middle of nowhere because a chain was loose or a bolt was coming undone then I could easily break a leg or hit my head, and I'd be done for.

Then I had the additional problem of having dementia, my toughest enemy yet, which made me even more paranoid about my kit. The Army had taught me strategies to think logically and remain vigilant. We were taught the metaphor 'if you keep tripping over, check your shoelaces'. So I did, figuratively speaking. There was no doubt that I was getting increasingly confused, though, especially about lefts and rights. I also had major blanks with place names as I tried to follow my route on my app or a map.

'How do you spell that?' I'd ask Vicks time and again, as she yawned back at me at some god-forsaken hour of the morning.

'It's called Snag Creek ... Sierra-November-

Alpha-Golf,' she'd reply, patiently spelling it out phonetically. Realising from my silence that I still hadn't grasped it, she'd encourage me, 'Think of each letter individually.'

The scary part was that most of the time I had no idea of my exact location or even what day it was. With few points of reference and nothing to gauge the days by, I hadn't a clue any more if it was a Sunday or a Wednesday, or even what month it was. My sense of dislocation from reality worsened if I was fatigued, so I found myself stopping people along the way to ask, 'Can you tell me where I am, please?' They must have thought I was mad, which I suppose wasn't that far from the truth.

Fortunately, I had my innate sense of humour to fall back on, something that had been actively encouraged in the British Army. Laughing things off had stood me in good stead over the years and would become of vital importance in the years to come. It was especially important when I was promoted to the rank of staff sergeant, with all its additional responsibilities. I'd loved being a full-screw – a corporal – because I was still one of the lads and didn't have too much else to think about. As a staff sergeant, I felt far less carefree so I'd get around it by putting people at their ease with humour. But to be funny you need to have someone to be funny with, and it felt strange and unusual on the road without that constant camaraderie and feedback. Vicks and I always had a good banter but the trouble was she knew all my corny jokes.

Out on the road hour after hour alone with my

mind was a kind of No Man's Land of its own – an indeterminate wasteland between two points. It was a limbo where humour didn't help and I couldn't help but reflect on the best and the worst parts of my life. My greatest regret by far was not being a better father to Natalie, who was born in 1999 shortly before I was sent to Kosovo, and Marcus, who was born in 2001 just before I was sent to Bahrain. I'd met their mother Kimmy in Norway early in 1998 when I was sent there for Arctic warfare training with the Allied Command Europe Mobile Force-Land or AMF(L). During my second winter tour of Norway in 1999, I married her.

Kimmy was originally from South Korea and had been adopted by a Norwegian family. We were crazy about each other from the start but not long after we met I was sent to Kosovo for six months. Then, the day after we married, I was sent to Bosnia for the same period. As I repeatedly travelled abroad she became what's known in the Army as a 'winter wife' – who only sees her husband for three or four months each year. Although she had her adoptive family nearby for support, that can't have been easy for a new bride and mother with a newborn.

I loved being in the Army so passionately that I have to confess I almost always put my career first. There wasn't anything else I wanted to do with my life or was even prepared to consider. For the next seven years Kimmy was left largely on her own, first in Norway and then at my base in South Cerney, while I served in Bahrain, the Balkans, Afghanistan and Italy. Our relationship became increasingly strained and we eventually separated in 2006, when I was in Germany and the kids were seven and six, divorcing a year later. It was a deeply unhappy time for us all and for a while I felt as if my whole world had collapsed. Not long afterwards, I accepted a tour to the Falkland Islands for nine months to try to sort my head out.

Being an incurable romantic, I met someone again not long after I returned to the UK. After another whirlwind romance we married in the summer of 2011. Once more, we didn't see that much of each other because I was sent on tour to Sierra Leone for two years, and the bulk of our relationship was conducted via Skype. We saw each other whenever I came home on leave but that was never going to be enough. Then I was sent to Kathmandu in Nepal, which was the first place we ever lived together, but we separated in early 2013. That was an equally unhappy time, and to try to clear my head again I took some leave.

By the time I met Vicky a year later in 2014, I was ready to risk love again. What I didn't know was how much she would come to mean to me, and to my future. Ironically, we discovered that our paths had first crossed in 1993 in Abingdon when I was eighteen years old and still a virgin. Her father was a former staff sergeant in bomb disposal who'd been based a few miles away in Didcot.

She and I ended up at the Black Swan pub, known locally as 'The Mucky Duck'. I spotted her across the crowded bar and couldn't take my eyes off her as I leaned against the fruit machine trying desperately to look cool. Vicky, who at nineteen was far more mature than I was and living in her own flat, took one look at me before turning to her friend and saying, 'What's he gawking at?' When I didn't look away, she thought I was just plain weird and said, 'When the bloody hell did this become a youth centre?' She never spoke one word to me but, apparently, my face was imprinted on her mind and she never forgot me.

More than twenty years later, after we finally reconnected at a military leaving do, she trawled through my old photos and was shocked to realise I was the same spotty young kid who'd yearned to chat her up all those years ago. As Vicks says, 'We'd been one step away from each other and the irony is that we could have had twenty years together – instead of just a handful.'

Regardless of the future, we were both determined from the outset to make the most of whatever time we had. As I made my way slowly west towards Anchorage and then Vancouver to meet up with the love of my life, I realised that the mere thought of seeing her again (and tasting some of her fantastic cooking) was what had kept me turning my wheels for the last 4,300 miles.

I only hoped she wouldn't mind my altered appearance. I must have lost about ten pounds in weight, my lips were blistered from the sun and I had white rings around my eyes from my sunglasses. I looked completely stupid naked, with a deep tan on my lower arms and legs only. The rest of me was as white as could be, covered in insect bites, with some unattractive rashes from sweating and chafing. Plus, I stank most of the time. My clothes were rank too, as they were only ever washed out with shampoo in campsite showers or sinks and then put back on wet. To top it all, my hair had grown too long, so I'd stopped at a barber's shop and asked for an extreme cut because of the heat. Perversely, I'd grown a small moustache and a goatee beard. On the rare occasions I caught a glimpse of myself in a mirror I noted with shock that I was no longer the handsome young toy boy she'd first fallen for.

There was nothing for it but to crack on as I approached the tiny town of Destruction Bay, aptly named for the damage the wind does to buildings there. With the US border a few miles up ahead of me there was no time to consider my looks, as I was too busy being stunned by the incredible views. One of my regrets about my life in the Army was that I didn't take enough photographs of the beautiful scenery I'd witnessed along the way. Even though stopping on my ride to capture yet another moment slowed me down, I couldn't help myself. I was traversing some of the most scenic routes in the world and the sweeping trans-Rockies highways were incredible.

The views of glaciers and mountains near Kluane Lake and National Park were by far the most spectacular I'd come across yet. It would have been criminal not to pause and be humbled by the sheer scale of the mountains. There was still a lot of snow on the peaks but it was the deep aquamarine hues of the lake that were so stunning. I don't think I'd ever seen water that colour before – but then I wouldn't remember if I had, would I?

A few miles further up, after a leg-sapping climb, the sweeping landscapes became even more astonishing. I rounded one corner and found the whole of the valley laid out before me. It was off-the-scale spectacular. 'Wow, Shirley!' I exclaimed, breathlessly. 'Take a look at that!' I climbed on and up through a place called Snag Junction and then to Beaver Creek, Canada's most westerly community, where I took a cheeky selfie by the town sign and posted it online. It sparked a few naughty comments from my mates until Vicky interjected with, 'Gentlemen, please. There are ladies present!'

Not much more than a hamlet populated by people from the White River First Nation, Beaver Creek had a little tin church and a café named Buckshot Betty's where I stopped for some scoff before checking into the only campsite. Annoyingly, it was Mozzie Central and I was eaten alive. I also suffered my first theft there – disappointingly at the hands of a fellow camper.

As always when I arrived anywhere, I went over to say hello the minute I spotted the young foreign cyclist travelling in the opposite direction to me. We chatted briefly, even though his English wasn't great, and I soon established that we were the only two campers. I noticed that he took a keen interest in my rig. Needing a good wash, I locked up Shirley and wandered to the shower block, taking my most valuable items with me as usual. Whenever I was in the loo, taking a shower, having dinner or asleep in my tent I had no choice but to rely on the honesty of those who could rifle through my panniers and steal my food and water while my back was turned.

When I emerged from the shower, I was surprised to see my campmate cycling off. It took me a few minutes to realise that he'd taken my waterproof poncho with him. This was an invaluable aid, brought with me all the way from the UK, that I used to cover my tent during downpours, keep the sun off during a heat wave, or pull over Shirley and me to protect us from the wind. I was so angry it had been stolen that I almost considered chasing after the thieving weasel as he headed east. Thinking more sensibly, though, I knew I could find myself in trouble if I confronted him and he denied it, so I elected to push on to the US border instead. In the end, I managed to find a hardware store that sold me a waterproof lightweight blanket that did an even better job than the poncho, so I decided to be grateful that the original had been pinched.

That wasn't the first time I'd been robbed, after all. I'd been charged over a hundred bucks a night to stay in some dives that made my childhood home in Eaton Road look like Buckingham Palace. At one remote spot near the Rockies I was staggered that the owners dared charge seventy-five dollars for a dirty, smelly cabin. I was even more disappointed to discover that there were no other guests, few facilities, no phone signal and no breakfast. The owner and his wife were really creepy too. He begrudgingly gave me the Wi-Fi code but then when I started chatting to Vicks online, he banged on my door and started bollocking me for using it. Not that I listened.

Then, without warning, at 10 p.m. he switched off the electricity so there were no lights, nothing. I thought he and his oddball wife were going to come and murder me in my bed so I went to bolt my door, to discover that it could only be locked from the outside. Alarmed, I wedged Shirley up against it in case they, or more worryingly a bear, came in while I was sleeping. I kept my torch close by me all night. Not surprisingly, I hardly slept and slipped away well before dawn.

I'd have been better off wild camping than wasting my money on such a shit-hole. I was getting pretty good at sleeping rough by then anyway, and had learned how to select the perfect location and then wait until dark because in most places overnight camping wasn't allowed. At a Timmy Horton's one night I set up my tent right by the bins at the back just to be able to access their free Wi-Fi. I was never chased off from places like that because I was quiet and the proprietors didn't even know I was there, plus I always set off before light. I knew my military stealth training would pay off in the end.

Move fast and stay low.

Vicks continued to be my mainstay back home and it became increasingly important to me to hear her voice at least once a day. How she continued to manage my needs as well as Dexter and Katy's, I'll never know. Plus, she was constantly answering messages from friends and family and keeping everyone up to speed. On 16 July she did her hair and make-up and posted a video from 'Mission Control' to show my growing numbers of followers how she was helping me. 'Chris and I thought it would be cool for you guys to see where it all happens, where all the planning gets done, how Chris manages to get from A to B and find accommodation, et cetera,' she said, beaming into the camera. 'I'm here every night, usually up until about two or three a.m. Tonight I shall be bedding down about three because he is due to land at one or two o'clock.'

She panned around to show the laptop that plotted my route and the terrain, and the second with my tracker details so she could log in and see where I was. From that she'd cut and paste my latitude and longitude on to a Google map to get my exact coordinates so she could figure out what lay up ahead. 'It looks like Chris is on a fairly easy one today – five hours, fifty miles,' she added wryly. 'He is set to land in Anchorage tomorrow or the day after, so that's all really exciting. Hopefully everything will go well for him today and I'm keeping my fingers crossed he won't go missing, which he has done on a few occasions. So, I'll be here just in case there's a problem with the campsite or the weather and he needs to find something closer or more suitable. Those of you going to bed in the next couple of hours, spare some zeds for me because it's going to be another long evening. Over and out.'

My sister Angie commented, 'For someone who's had so little sleep, you look fab! You are both doing brill and like everyone has said it takes a special lady to do what you do. Big thank you.' Our youngest sibling Lizzie added, 'It's fab that Chris has someone so supportive at the end of the phone when he needs to sort accommodation urgently.' Someone else thanked Vicks for 'keeping the brave little focker safe', while others claimed we both 'deserved a medal' or that Vicky was the great woman behind the man. Never a truer word was spoken.

Although getting to Anchorage had been such a major goal during the previous two months, if I'm honest it was a bit of an anti-climax once I arrived. Having left the good people of Canada behind me on 12 July, I'd cycled across thirty or so miles of no man's land comprising open tundra and swamp between the two countries before reaching the US border near the town of Northway Junction. Once there, the border guard insisted on going through all my paperwork with a fine-tooth comb.

'Where are you going and what are your plans while in the United States?' he asked me with something approaching a growl. I played the game and answered all his questions, being careful to call him 'sir', but he reminded me of the worst kind of camp guard as he checked and triple-checked my visa and every other document. He had a little bit of power and he was determined to use it.

When I eventually reached my hostel in Anchorage four hundred miles later on 20 July, it was quite a shock as there were so many down-and-outs and such a marked contrast between the rich and the poor. The whole place seemed rather shabby, chiefly because so many of the Native Americans and Alaskan Natives seemed to live in abject poverty at the lower end of the social scale.

Having grown up in Bowdon Vale, I knew what

it felt like to be poor, hungry and underprivileged, so wherever I was sent on tour during my military career, I always tried to do what I could to help out those less fortunate than I was. Mostly, it was about giving someone a few extra quid or sneaking them some food, as we did in Bosnia and Sierra Leone. I'd also take time out to train up anyone who wanted to join the army and pass the fitness tests, and I taught loads of kids in Nepal how to play football. In Liberia, I even taught the coastguards how to swim, which was potentially life saving when their boats were far from seaworthy.

It was when I was based in war-ravaged Sierra Leone in 2009-11, however, that I decided to go the extra mile. Every time I visited a favourite café in the capital, Freetown, I'd bump into a young man named Jib. He was probably about nineteen but it was impossible to tell as everyone there looked old before their time. Desperately poor, he'd offer to park our car for us and then guard it against theft in return for a few *leones,* the local currency. Jib was one of the many victims of the eleven-year civil war that had virtually destroyed his nation. The task of our unit out there was to train up the local police and do what we could to maintain a tenuous peace. It was a beautiful country with fantastic people and stunning beaches but the place was in ruins.

'Where do you live, Jib?' I asked the local boy one day.

'In the slums, like everyone else.'

'Will you show me?'

He looked at me as if I was mad, but a few days

later I asked again and he eventually took me to the shantytown on the beach where he shared a one-room corrugated tin shack with his grand-mother, two other siblings and a family friend. They had no toilet and shared an outside tap with their many neighbours. Even though there was such limited space between them, their home was piled to its leaky ceiling with old, rotting clothes and it reeked.

'Flipping heck, Jib!' I cried. 'What are all these clothes doing here?'

He looked embarrassed and pointed at his grandmother, who I suspect was a few pence short of a *leone*. He explained that she collected and hoarded clothes. I suggested quietly that he dispose of them as soon as he could, as they were a serious health hazard.

Having seen what a horrible tip they were living in, I knew immediately that I could do something about it using some of the extra salary I received for being in Sierra Leone. As soon as I left the shantytown, I drove straight round to a local hardware store owned by an ex-Army mate and asked him to order me in some supplies. 'I'll need some zinc, timber and nails. Oh, and can you recommend a local carpenter please?' He asked me what I was doing so I told him, but I didn't want it too widely known so he promised not to say anything. The local builder he recommended was enthusiastic and honest and agreed to start work the following week. I went back to see Jib the day before work was due to begin and was annoyed to find the place was still stacked high with even more stinking clothes.

'Please explain to your grandmother that I'm going to build her a new house,' I told him in frustration. 'We need to clear all this stuff out.' Picking up some of it, I started hurling it into a pile outside the door to demonstrate how it could be done. She protested and complained but Jib was clearly relieved. He explained that she was anxious that I might start something I wouldn't finish and leave them homeless, but I assured them that the job would be done in three days.

It was only when we knocked down their shack and laid a new concrete base that they believed I was serious. Within three days they were able to move back into a brand new home with a sound floor, substantial walls, sturdy poles and a new roof. I even found them some old Army beds with rubber mattresses so they no longer had to sleep on the dirt. To change these people's lives cost me a little over £1,000. By the time it was finished it looked really good and they were clearly grateful.

Job done. Or was it?

Six months later I went back to visit them during the rainy season, naïvely expecting to find them living happily ever after. I should have known better than to hope for a fairytale ending. To begin with, the family didn't exactly welcome me with open arms and I soon realised why. One of their neighbours had become so jealous of their new home that he'd attacked it with rocks. One boulder he'd hurled at it had created a huge hole in the roof, which had clearly been there for some time. It was leaking water directly over one of the new beds, which was now rendered use-less.

'Jib!' I cried. 'Why the hell didn't you move that bed three inches out of the way?'

He looked at me with the kind of expression that made me feel like Einstein. Trying not to judge him, I patched the roof and then went to visit the troublesome neighbour. I told him in no uncertain terms that if I heard he'd done anything like that again, I'd be round with some of my mates to sort him out.

My experiences with that family in Sierra Leone proved to be a salutary lesson. I discovered there that you can only help people so much and sometimes when you try to do something good it has unforeseen consequences that can end up making matters worse. Foolishly, it didn't occur to me that Jib's neighbours would be driven crazy with envy over what they'd been given. Or that he and his grandmother would stick to their way of life regardless of my intervention.

There are probably many people in Canada and the US who do what they can to help the First Nation families that live in their midst and, who knows, maybe it backfires on them sometimes too. I knew from my own experiences that I shouldn't judge. But I also knew that it was a real eye opener seeing so many hard-up people in Anchorage and along my route there, and it made me even keener to get south to my little family as soon as I could.

If in doubt – get out.

8

'Whatever the mind can conceive and believe, the mind can achieve.'

NAPOLEON HILL

Dementia Adventure Diary, 20 August 2015, Sumas, Washington State

One of the hardest legs of my entire charity bike ride was starting again after my glorious time off with Vicky and Dexter in Vancouver. It was horrible to say goodbye to them – plus I had to retrain my body and reset my muscle memory all over again.

Not that I'd have missed seeing them for the world. Once I'd finally made it to that stunning city on the bay it was fantastic to take a break and catch up with 'the boss' and our little monster. I was so ready to see them and felt surprisingly emotional at having them both back in my arms.

Vicky was pleased to see me too, even though we very nearly had a bust-up over which route I took to make our rendezvous on time. The problem was that I refused to use boats, trucks, buses or planes unless I had no other choice. Mine was a one-man endurance challenge and I intended to cycle myself the whole way round from start to finish, even if it meant going back over the same route. This plan ran into major problems, however, especially after I insisted on cycling all the way to Anchorage from Calgary because, unbeknown to me, there were no direct routes south once I got there. Incredibly, more than half of the coastline of the United States is in Alaska because it has so many inlets and bays. Traversing it by bike was a no go, especially with Vicky and Dexter arriving in six days' time.

This meant that by the time I reached Anchorage I had only a few options left. There wasn't a direct train route either and in any case, the railway company refused to take Shirley any distance. That left a choice of flying to Vancouver, boarding a ferry from the small port of Whittier, Alaska, or hiring a car. Whichever I chose I'd still have to get back to Calgary after Vicks flew home so that I could pick up the route where I left off. That would be the only way to keep a continuous link in the chain.

'But Chris, if you do that it'll mean you'll have to cross the Rockies again!' she reminded me. 'And you've already cycled all the way to the Gulf of Alaska, so it's not like you can be accused of slacking!'

'I don't care,' I replied stubbornly. 'I don't want anyone to accuse me of cheating. I have to do this properly or not at all.'

When we looked at all the different costings for getting to Vancouver it was clear the cheapest option by far would have been to hire a car. Annoyingly that wasn't possible for me because my driving licence, which had to be renewed annually because of my dementia, had expired in June. Annual testing is standard procedure for someone with my condition, so each year the DVLA liaises with my doctors to establish if I need an assessment by an instructor sitting alongside me while I drive. Only then do they decide. When I left the UK, I didn't imagine that I might need a current driving licence, but in Alaska it became a massive inconvenience and completely ruled out the possibility of hiring a car.

Unable to find myself another 'Mindy' to drive Shirley and me south, I had no choice but to go for the second cheapest option with all my kit and take a short train ride to Whittier, sixty miles away. From there I boarded a ferry for the five-day, 2,200-mile journey south, getting me into Vancouver less than twenty-four hours before Vicks arrived. Shockingly, the steerage ticket set me back C$600 and that didn't even include the luxury of a bunk, plus I had no choice on board but to pay premium rates for all my meals. Instead of a proper bed, I had to sleep 'for free' on an unforgiving wooden lounger on the sundeck with a couple of hardy backpackers. They were pleasant enough company, but I was bored shitless and restless as hell after almost seven thousand miles under my belt. Worst of all there was no telly, which meant no footy!

Savages. Didn't they know who I was?

In spite of my cheerful daily updates online, I was actually in a bit of a pickle by then because – with all these extra costs – my funds were running out. There was a real chance that I might not be able to complete my ride and if that happened, I would have been gutted, and Vicks too. I tried to make savings wherever I could, but my food bill

143

alone was almost £100 a day at times and even if I camped each night, we were running on empty. For a while I set the tracker to only ping every few hours to save money but that freaked Vicky out too much because she didn't know where I was, so we put it back to the regular setting.

My mate Pete Davies stepped into the breach in a magnificent way. A few days after I left Whittier, he organised a sponsored run for me from my old barracks at South Cerney. He managed to rally nineteen lads and lasses to take part in the Cotswolds 24-Hour Race in relays of 9 km laps the day before Vicks flew to Canada. She piled Dexter and Katy in the car, and joined my sister Lizzie and her fella Kev on the run after they'd driven from Manchester to take part as well. I'm sure it almost broke them physically but, together, they raised a much-needed £1,500 to cover my costs.

As I told them all on the sitrep video I posted that day: 'I'd like to say a massive, massive thank you to Pete Davies and all the people who are doing a charity run this weekend coming. Massive respect. I appreciate it. If I could do the run with you, you know I would. But take your time at it. Keep yourself hydrated and you'll be fine.'

As I waited for our 'dinghy' to arrive in Whittier, I added, 'Me and Shirley will hopefully have our sea legs and won't puke too much... Hopefully we won't be sunk in the sea somewhere and we'll speak soon. If in doubt, in this case – paddle!'

Seeing Vicky's smiling face when I went to meet them at Vancouver airport a few days later was well worth all the hassle. I couldn't get over how thin she was though – she'd lost three stone and all her

144

baby weight in the three months since I'd been gone. One of her first comments when she saw me was, 'You're still in your cycling shorts!' She, of all people, knew I didn't have anything other than Lycra to wear (which is why she'd brought me an extra large case with regular clothing for our holiday), although I suppose I could have put my longer keks on.

The weather was beautifully sunny and warm for their visit and we'd rented the lower floor of a house in Moody Avenue, North Vancouver. We went out to see the famous beluga whales at the aquarium, but we didn't do much more sightseeing because Dex was proper moody with jet lag. Neither of us minded – we were happy just to spend time in each other's company. I was amazed by how big Dexter had grown in the three months I'd been away and how much he looked like me, poor little bugger. Vicky has since come across some old photos of me at the same age and he's the spitting image of me, right down to the same cheeky expressions and mannerisms.

One of our favourite photographs of the three of us was taken in Vancouver, and when we posted it online we were inundated with comments, wishing us all the best and delighted we were having 'precious time together'. It really was precious, but like all good things it flew by.

Before I knew it, 8 August had come around and our holiday was over. As my lovely little family headed for the airport to jump ship back to Blighty, I was on the road again with fresh legs. This time it was in a Greyhound bus heading back towards Calgary and the home of a friend of

Dean Stokes who'd kindly agreed to put me up for a night or two. I'd stayed with former Para Frank Henvey on my way west and when I rang him up out of the blue again and asked for a bed, he said, 'Yeah, sure. Come on Gurkhs!' with the same kind of open friendliness I'd encountered throughout. He and his wife Pascale booked Shirley in for a service, threw me a barbecue and introduced me to their friends, filling me with food and setting me up nicely for the next leg, where I'd be climbing to more than five thousand feet – again!

Traversing the Rockies was brutal and my legs felt far from fresh. In fact my pedalling lost its symmetry for a while and I found it hard to find my rhythm. It was hot and sticky, so I was de-hydrating so much through sweating that there were times when I longed to stop and drink my supplies dry. The salt in my sweat was stinging my eyes and dripping off my face, and I had a throbbing ache in my hamstrings. This was a real test of my mental and physical stamina.

Athletes often talk about 'hitting the wall' and the need to push on past that point but I'd never really experienced it up until then. Even when I ran a marathon from base camp at Mount Everest while I was based in Kathmandu, I hadn't found it that hard. Admittedly, I had some breathing diffi-culties at 16,500 feet and it wasn't easy carrying six kilos of safety equipment with oxygen in short supply. There was a lot of ice on the ground and the terrain up and down over the mountain trails was extremely rough. Fifteen of us, including some genuine Gurkhas, ran the twenty-six miles in pairs from Gorak Shep close to base camp until we reached the Sherpa town of Namche Bazaar. I came in first at six hours eight minutes with my partner-in-crime Mark Black. And best of all – we beat the Gurkhas.

Let's be having you!

Far tougher than that was a marathon I ran in Rome in 2004 after two weeks of downhill skiing. This was during my two-year posting in beautiful Milan with NATO and the British Consulate (where, strangely, everyone from my mum to Neil to Lizzie came to visit me). Foolishly, I'd been out on the beer the previous night and felt as rough as anything that morning. I honestly thought I might die. I missed the start of the race because I was puking so much and I was moving more like an old man than an athlete. Somehow I got round the course and managed to finish it in just under four hours, but that was the closest to the 'wall' I've ever been. I don't recommend running a marathon without any training as a hangover cure.

Cycling the Rockies I was in a different kind of pain. My legs were screaming, the steep climbs played havoc with my dodgy knee, and I was back to www.sorebum.com. It was soon after that when I found out that I needed to adjust my seat and handlebars to a better angle. Vicks had Googled my problem for me, and a local bike shop gave me some additional advice. Once I'd made the relevant alterations, my knee squared itself away again.

Although the weather was a bit too hot for cycling up mountains, at least there was no wind to dry out my mouth or blast grit into my eyes.

And there were far fewer bugs at that altitude, so I was grateful for small mercies. I tried to persuade myself that the Rockies weren't as big as they appeared. Crossing them was definitely testing. The roads between the peaks were incredibly winding with loads of hairpin bends, so drivers would only spot Shirley and me as they rounded a corner. They'd veer so close that I'd sometimes have to stop just to save myself from getting mowed down.

On one corner I came face to face with a speeding lorry on my side of the road. There was nowhere to go so I had to make a snap decision. I threw myself off the bike and landed hard on a steep slope, which hurt like hell. The lorry didn't even slow down. Tunnels were equally dangerous, even though I had lights front and back, because drivers would race up behind me at speed and only see me at the last minute. I think I came off at least twice on that leg of the journey and I had the bruises to prove it.

At my much-needed next rest stop in Lake Louise in Banff National Park, I was finally able to relax. I posted a video to show off my smart campground, surrounded by an electric fence to stop the bears getting in. I panned the camera round to Shirley and my tent, which was pitched next to those belonging to a bunch of friendly Swedish cyclists.

Looking back on that footage now, it's obvious how much of a boost it had given me to see Vicky and Dex and have some quality time together. Despite the tough climbs I'd faced and had yet to come, I look positively chipper. I loved it every time 'Happy' by Pharrell Williams came around on my playlist, because that's exactly how I felt then. *Can't nothing bring me down because my level's too high,* I sang along, and I wasn't talking about the altitude.

It must have been that new energy that helped me press on, up and over the mountains, and down towards the American border. By 20 August I was still in great spirits as I entered a town called Hope where I posted a photo with the caption, 'Where there is Hope, there is a cure for dementia.' Later that day I finally crossed the border.

'Phase 2 of the Long Cycle Round commencing soon!' Vicky posted excitedly, and it certainly felt significant to cycle into Washington State from British Columbia at a place called Sumas, crossing the longest international border in the world. 'It's downhill all the way from there!' one of my followers quipped, and it did feel important psychologically to be out of the headwinds and facing south.

Vicks was great at keeping my morale up with her cheery chatter in my ear and was the first to lightheartedly accuse me of being a 'slacker' if my mileage was less than expected. As Neil Deadman once correctly declared, 'Most of Chris's relationships are based on good-humoured banter and abuse.' Sometimes even for me, though, it was tough to remain in a positive frame of mind when the elements were against me. If I didn't push through the miles and make enough progress each day then that would definitely affect my mood. I needed to achieve a big chunk of the distance daily, not just because I'd got it into my head quite early on that I wanted to be home for Dexter's first Christmas, but because I knew I was running out of money again – and that was panicking me big time.

I had to finish this. I had to get all the way round. It was the one thing that I'd set myself to achieve and whatever else lay ahead of me I needed to do this.

Until fairly recently, I wasn't the sort of bloke who'd even know what was good or bad for me psychologically. I was the kind of person who didn't think too much about anything if I could help it and just got on with life. As long as I was able to go for my daily run, come home, shower, eat, do something productive, and have the love of a good woman, I was happy.

All of that changed in about 2008 when my world started to fall apart. I can't quite remember who told me first, but it was almost certainly my sister Lizzie in one of our regular phone calls. She had become my unofficial PA over the years, sending me anything I needed from the UK to wherever I was based, and phoning up to let me know another parcel was on its way. During one of our hour-long chats, she told me that she feared that our brother Anthony was starting to develop dementia as he kept repeating himself and forgetting things.

I could hardly believe it. Tony? The big bro who'd always been so fiercely independent, going his own way, treading his own path? It didn't seem that long ago that I'd driven to see him in Newport in my clapped-out Ford Orion – frightening the life out of Neil with my driving in the worst rain we'd ever seen. Tony was always pleased to see me and the feeling was happily mutual. After his dud start to life, he'd become a hard-working family man of faith and someone who'd proudly stepped in for Dad to give Lizzie away when she got married in Cyprus.

Admittedly, he'd not quite been himself in recent years and had shocked everyone by un-expectedly leaving Jan, his wife of thirteen years, for his childhood sweetheart Jayne, who was pregnant with his first child. He moved back to Manchester with her and they went on to have two lovely sons, Richard and James. In spite of the massive change of circumstances, he secured himself a great new managerial position with a big vehicle auction company in Leeds and was thrilled to be a dad.

Although I'd not seen so much of him or his new family in recent years, we'd always grab a few scoops or a full English breakfast together when-ever I was home. We'd become far closer than we'd ever been in childhood and had a right laugh together. The thought of him being anything other than fully able-bodied and sharp-witted was devastating. Soon after I learned of his predica-ment, I flew home to go on a course and went straight round to his house, taking Neil with me.

'How's it going, bro?' I asked, and Tony replied that he was fine apart from the headaches he'd been having. 'Have you managed to get to any footy games lately?' I enquired, keeping the con-versation deliberately light. We chewed the fat as normal and to begin with I was relieved because I couldn't see any major difference in him. Then he asked us if we wanted something to drink.

'You know me, Tone. I'd love a cup of tea,' I replied. 'Two sugars please.'

He wandered out of the room but a few minutes later he was back in. 'Can I get you something to drink?'

'Yes, Tony. A cup of tea with two sugars,' I said, the hairs rising on the back of my neck. He must have asked us four times before he finally got it and then my brew arrived with no sugar at all. I knew then that something was wrong. The next time I flew home, Neil and I took Tony to the pub where he started drinking whisky. He seemed depressed, and after thirty minutes he was so drunk we had to take him home. I don't think he could handle alcohol any more and he started to go downhill after that.

I may be a sandwich short of a picnic, but even at that point I didn't think his condition had anything to do with me. Maybe I was just playing ostrich again, but nor did I relate it directly to the death of our father. After all, Dad had died in a loony bin, hadn't he? Water on the brain, they'd said. What did that have to do with Tony or me? I was astonished to discover years later that Tony knew exactly what Dad died of and had always been fearful of developing similar symptoms. His wife Jan revealed that even before they were married, he'd gone for some medical tests to make sure there was nothing wrong with him and was so relieved when the results came back that he was normal.

'Tony remembered the men coming to take his father away,' she said. 'He'd started to research the

Graham history for a family tree and became extremely emotional if he came across any photos of his dad. We even talked about adopting if it turned out that he'd inherited the disease too, but then we didn't have children anyway.'

Not that long after Tony moved back to Manchester, he developed the terrible headaches he described as 'like something crawling around inside my skull'. In the following few years these got worse, and then he started to be affected in other ways. He had momentary lapses of attention that gave him problems driving and trouble with spatial awareness that meant he kept pranging his car. His speech changed and he sometimes didn't make sense. He found it difficult to use technology and then he started having seizures. Eventually his driving licence was taken away and he had to give up work. Even then, he showed the Graham determination and started building a conservatory at home.

Jan is a truly godly woman. Incredibly, she forgave Tony for leaving her and remained in close contact with him and Jayne, who had to work full-time to provide for her family. Jan even offered respite care once Tony became seriously unwell, taking him back to their old marital home in Wales one weekend in every month. She never remarried or found someone else to share her life with. 'I love being with Tony and taking care of him whenever I can, even though it soon became a bit like looking after a child,' she said.

Like me, my brother always enjoyed his food and had a healthy appetite. 'He had the happiest expressions whenever he was eating,' Jan added, 'or when I took him to the local farm to see the animals. We'd link arms and run down the hill together like we were kids.' To this day she still visits him every week and has continued to support Jayne and the boys.

Before Tony was unable to communicate with us any more, he let us all know that not only had he been diagnosed with early-onset Alzheimer's at the same age as Dad, but that each of us had a 50/50 chance of developing it too. Poor Lizzie was in tears after learning this on her second daughter's first birthday, which was also the day Bella was christened.

'Tony was really quiet that day and he kept forgetting Bella's name and referring to her as a boy, so I asked him what was wrong. That's when he blurted it out,' she said. 'He seemed to have taken the diagnosis quite well and told me, "I'm the eldest. I *should* get it." We were having a party with loads of friends and family and I was really shocked and had to hold it together. I kept thinking about Bella and wishing I'd known two years earlier.'

I was based in South Cerney when Lizzie phoned and I finally realised the serious implications for the rest of us, and for all of our children. It was such a painful time for the whole family and I didn't think any of us really knew how to handle the information at first. I know I didn't. I felt vulnerable and frightened and wanted to get away. When I remembered that Neil was travelling on his own around Australia and New Zealand for several months, I took five weeks' 'renewal leave', known as REN leave, and flew out to join him. I packed my tent and my Jetboil and we hired a car and drove around New Zealand together like the sad single blokes that we were.

When I eventually came home on leave I went to see Tony, who'd been referred to genetics specialists in Manchester and to the Dementia Research Unit in London. It was they who had first tested his DNA after they learned of Dad's diagnosis and the early deaths of our grandfather and aunt. That triggered the alarm bells, and they discovered a pattern of familial Alzheimer's disease, or FAD. I knew that Dad's father had died young, as had his sister Thelma, but in Tony's family research he discovered that Thelma's daughter Wendy had also died of dementia at an early age.

'It's in our genes, Chris,' he told me. 'There's only a few hundred families with this mutation in the whole world and we're among them.'

'How lucky are we?' I quipped, feeling sick.

His medical team urged that we all speak to a genetics counsellor at the Manchester Centre for Genomic Medicine. With her guidance we were asked to consider what this unwelcome inheritance might mean for us and our children, and to help us decide whether or not we wanted to be tested. This included questioning the implications of the result if it proved positive, what level of ongoing health and counselling support we might expect in the future, and what this could mean for any plans to have more children.

Lizzie wanted the test straight away to stop prolonging the agony, as she put it, but she was shown a graph, given some literature, and warned that once she knew the information it had the

155

potential to ruin her life. 'I so wanted to go ahead, but something the counsellor said really struck a chord. She said that as long as I didn't know I would always have hope. The moment I had the information no one would be able to take it back and – I couldn't cope – it could amount to a loss of hope. In the end, my husband persuaded me to walk away and not consider it again until the girls were of childbearing age.'

For the next four years Lizzie was convinced she was going to die young. 'Like Chris, I'd always been a bit dipsy and I began to blame every memory lapse on it to the point that it coloured everything about my life. I wrote memory books for the girls full of photographs and words of advice for after I'd died, and we specifically didn't have any more kids because we thought that would be irresponsible.'

My sister Angie felt much the same way, but she was adamant she didn't want the test. 'It was such a dilemma but I was sure I didn't want to know.' My sisters had always been much more decisive than me about the important things in life but I was a bit blasé and considered myself bulletproof.

'We're all going to die anyway,' I told them. 'Don't worry, if I find out I've got it I'm not going to say, "Now where's the rope?"'

If I'd been a betting man I'd have wagered that I definitely had the 'daft gene' lurking in me because I've never had the best memory in the world. I was often late (just like my dad) and frequently lost my keys, or forgot where I was meant to be. Once I learned the true nature of the threat hanging over us, everything suddenly made perfect sense. In a weird way, it came as a relief because it finally explained so much. I wasn't just thick after all.

Fall in, soldier.

I understood my sisters' very personal decision not to confirm the diagnosis and I totally sympathised, but I wanted to crack on. Because of my foreign tour and various other factors, though, the process took over a year. During that time I had several counselling consultations to check that I was strong enough to handle the news and to let me know what would happen if I chose to go ahead.

'I've made up my mind and I want to take the test,' I told them repeatedly. 'My dad and my grandad had it and my brother's got it, so I'd much rather know.' In spite of the fact that I was adamant throughout, they still needed to go through the procedures of asking questions and analysing my answers, which really started messing with my head. In the end, I couldn't bear to live with the 'what if?' any more. I've never been the kind of bloke to hide behind my hands in a horror movie. I'd be the first to say, 'Boo! Who's behind that door?'

It was time to say Boo.

By this time I'd divorced Kimmy and was dating again. I was still working in Africa and I needed to know one way or the other – not just for me but also for my children. What were we waiting for? It was only a simple blood test and then I could know what I was facing and maybe start on some treatment. 'I want to plan for the future,' I told the doctors. 'There's no point in hiding from it.' Besides, I'd been in the Army nearly twenty years and I fully expected them to help and support me physically, emotionally and financially to the end of my service – which meant that I'd be far better off than Tony, who was virtually unemployable by then.

Most of the colleagues I worked with in Sierra Leone knew what I was up against but I'd decided not to officially inform anyone in the Army hierarchy until I had the test results. I wasn't trying to hide anything but I figured there was no point alarming anybody unnecessarily, especially when I didn't believe that my few memory lapses affected my work in any way.

It was the summer of 2010 when I took some leave and flew home to Manchester to finally take the test. I watched the nurse siphon off a few phials of my blood, knowing that the worst part would be marking time until I knew the results. It was a month before I could get leave to fly home again, so I booked the hospital appointment for 12 October 2010, which – ironically – is Vicky's birthday, even though I hadn't met her (properly) yet. I walked into the counsellor's office, sat down and heard the doctor tell me, 'I'm sorry Chris, but you do have the mutation.'

Even though I was half-expecting it, the news that I carried the dementia gene still came as a body blow. Despite all my bravado, I wasn't nearly as prepared as I thought. I felt completely winded. I was also in such a strange place emotionally because I had Natalie and Marcus to think of too, as well as the new woman in my life.

The doctors tried to reassure me that even

though I'd tested positive they didn't believe I had any concerning symptoms yet. 'Keeping fit is the best possible thing you can do to remain well and you're in peak condition,' they added. 'Plus research is coming up with new solutions all the time...'

'What about my kids?' I interrupted, almost on autopilot.

'They now have a fifty-fifty chance of carrying the mutation too,' came the reply. I didn't break down exactly but my eyes definitely filled with tears at that point. I was barely able to take in the information that my two healthy teenagers might have to face the same shattering news one day.

'When can they be tested?' I asked, choked.

'Not until they're eighteen. It's a question of ethics. They have to be old enough to decide for themselves and mature enough to deal with the information.' Everyone did their best to reassure me that by the time they were in their thirties, when the symptoms usually begin, there would almost certainly be a cure. 'And if a cure is found before then, we'd expect that you'd be called in to trial it before anyone else.'

'And definitely before any Man City fans,' I quipped, desperately trying to recover myself.

I rang Lizzie from the hospital to tell her the news. 'I'd accepted it with Tony,' she told me, sobbing, 'but not you!' She could tell I was upset too but I refused to let her, or anyone else, see me cry. My testing positive only convinced her still further that she also had the 'daft gene', because we were so alike in every other way.

The next few months are a bit of a blur for me.

I can't honestly say that I knew what I was doing half the time with all the thoughts about my future spinning round and round in my head. My response to anything distressing has usually been to do something proactive, so in January 2011 I decided to climb Mount Kilimanjaro to raise money for Alzheimer's Research. I'd wanted to scale it ever since I'd been in Africa, so I suppose doing it then was my way of dealing with the information. When we were almost at the summit I suddenly proposed to my girlfriend and she accepted. Sadly, our marriage wasn't destined to last much longer than a year. Once again, I turned to the Army to save me from the harsher realities of life, although my family, friends and colleagues rallied around me in ways I could never have imagined.

It was while I was still out in Sierra Leone that I first watched the television programme that followed Mark Beaumont cycling the Americas. It was almost unthinkable that, having already broken the record for pedalling around the world, he would then cycle 13,000 miles through twelve countries and climb the continent's two highest peaks. Watching him on that incredible ride inspired me to come up with my own plan to follow his wheel tracks and make a few of my own, partially as a testament to the green beret I so proudly wore. I'd always wanted to take on a big sporting challenge to mark the end of my military career, and this seemed perfect.

My friends and family thought it was an unimaginable thing to do, given that I'd hardly ridden a bike before and was now facing a death sentence, but for me it seemed unimaginable not

My father John with
my brother Tony as
a baby in 1973

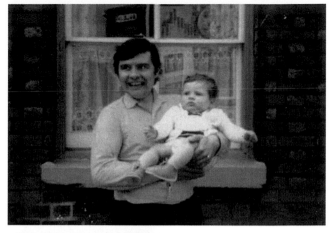

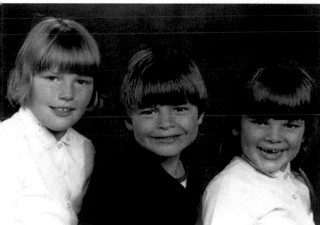

Angie, me and
Lizzie, school photo
circa 1981

Me in my school
uniform 1984

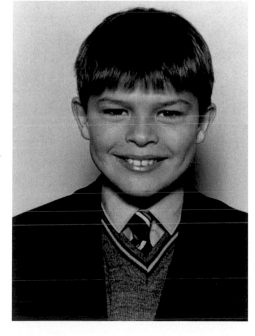

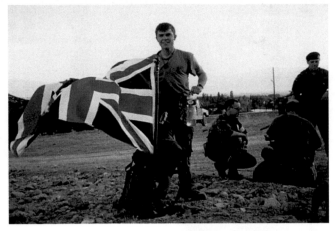

Proudly flying the Union Flag on a NATO exercise in Turkey, 1996

Me, bottom right, looking like Jai from Tarzan on a Devon exercise, 1994

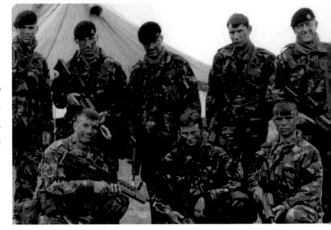

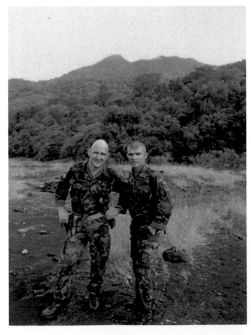

With my friend Dean Stokes in Sierra Leone, 2011

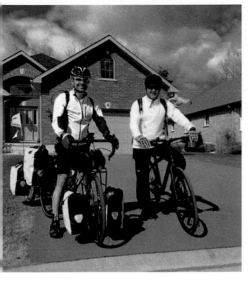

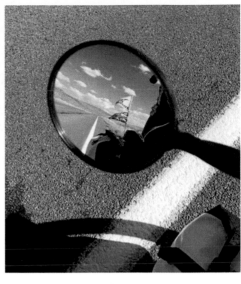

Setting off on my bike ride with Dean Stokes, April 2015, Brighton, Ontario

My rear view for the next 16,000 miles

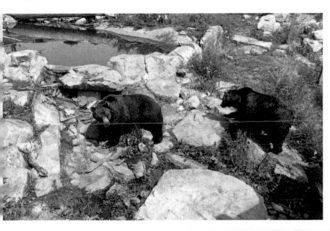

Black bears on the prowl in Canada

Visiting former colleagues at the BFPO in BATUS, Canada

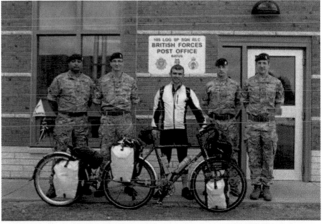

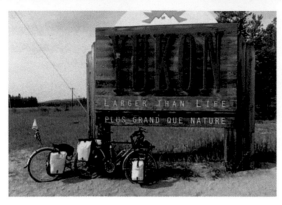

Crossing onto
Yukon Territory
– Larger than Life

Another day,
another mountain

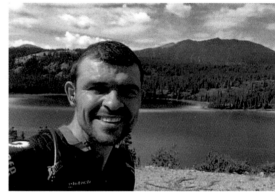

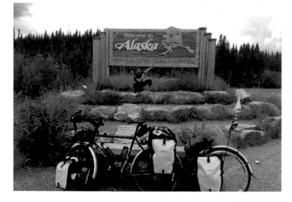

Crossing into Alaska
heading for my first
'corner' of North America

Hitching a ride on a boat
to meet up with my family
in Vancouver

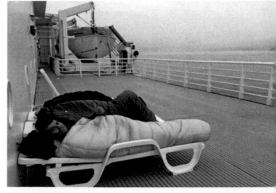

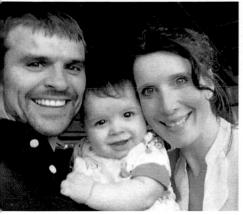

Happy to be reunited with
Vicks and Dexter

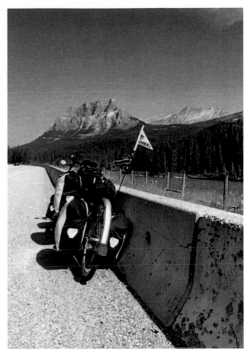

Ain't no mountain
high enough

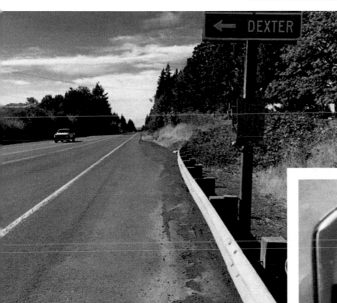

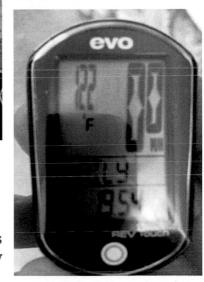

Quick detour to enjoy
Dexter, Oregon

122 degrees at almost 8pm as
I head towards Death Valley

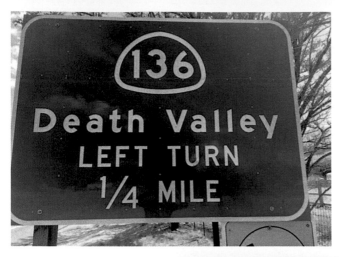

No turning back –
Death Valley

Still smiling despite
the heat, snakes and
scorpions

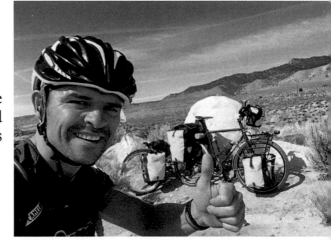

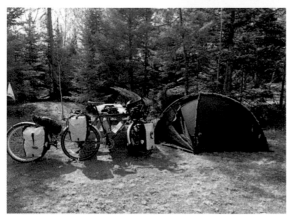

Wild camping by the side of the road

Typical pit-stop at Jawbone Canyon

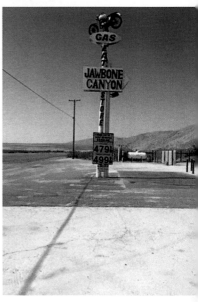

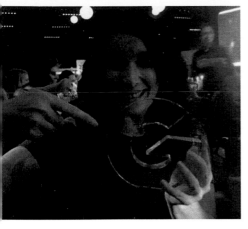

Vicky with my Just Giving
Endurance Award in London

Yet another
glorious sunrise

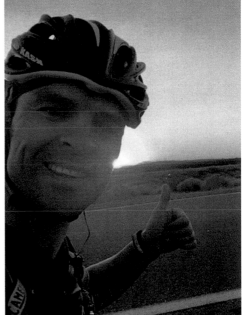

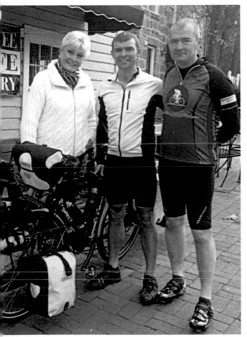

Filming the documentary with
Pete Davies and Angela
Rippon in Washington, DC

Only my shadow
for company

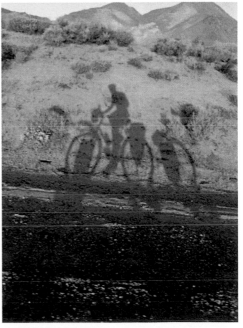

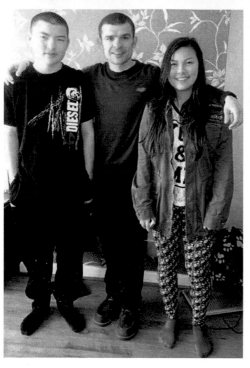

Proud father of Natalie
and Marcus

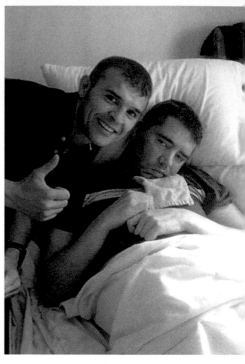

With my brother, Tony

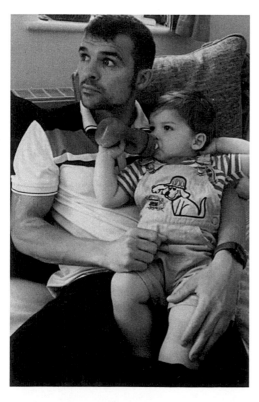

Wedding Day, June 2016.
'Til death us do part. . .

Hanging out with Dex

to at least attempt it.

Five years after I was first spurred into action, and as I continued to attempt the unthinkable, I was as keen as ever to prove to myself – and everyone else – that I was still capable of it. With at least 10,000 miles still to go it was time to stop dwelling on what I couldn't control and get on with what I could.

If in doubt – commando on.

9

'The only journey is the one within.'
RAINER MARIA RILKE

Dementia Adventure Diary, 3 September 2015, Oregon/California border

Once I'd put Canada behind me and was finally in what felt like the real United States (Alaska seemed almost identical to the Yukon), I was filled with sudden gratitude for how well I'd been treated so far.

Aside from the odd unscrupulous motel owner, most people had gone out of their way to welcome and care for me, inviting me into their tents, RVs, trucks and homes to make what I was doing just that little bit more bearable. Full of the milk of human kindness, I posted a sitrep on 29 August in which I began with my usual, 'Hello Dementia Adventure friends wherever you are in the world, I hope you are fine, well and most dandy.' In my update I expressed my thanks to all the Canadians and Alaskans for looking after me so well as I'd travelled through their land.

'You've all been fantastic. You've put me up, fed and watered me and helped me along the way and I won't forget that,' I told them. 'Clearly I will see the Canadian people again when I come back through Nova Scotia but I just wanted to thank everyone again for all the help they've given me.'

I was deeply touched by other acts of kindness too, including the sheer numbers of people who'd taken the time to vote for me in the 2015 Just Giving Endurance Fundraiser of the Year, which Alzheimer's Research had kindly nominated me for. With the slogan, 'Celebrating the people who make good things happen', the annual awards are given to eight fundraisers in categories including mine, as well as the Community Crowdfunder of the Year, Young Fundraiser of the Year, and Charity of the Year.

I was one of three finalists for the endurance award, the other two being James Latch, the father of a boy with cancer, who completed the London marathon and then ran home to Wales to raise £76,000 for charity. The other finalist was cystic fibrosis sufferer Emily Hoyle, who'd climbed the highest live volcano in the world to raise £23,000 for To Transplant and Beyond after she had a life-saving double lung transplant. I was in illustrious and humbling company and wished them both the best of luck.

Oregon is truly beautiful. It's known not only as 'The Beaver State' but also as the mountain biking capital of the north-west. After the Rockies, it was a pleasure to be cycling what felt like downhill, with no headwinds to batter my once flawless complexion. Instead, I could almost feel a whisper of a southern breeze. I was treated extremely well there too, and was even invited to sleep on the sofa in the kitchen of one generous bike-friendly guest-house owner who had nowhere else to put me.

It was still high season and the weather was good, so a lot of the campsites were full, or at best crowded. Vicky continued to navigate me brilliantly and get me safely to a different place each night, but sometimes this didn't go to plan. Somewhere between Portland and a town called Eugene at the end of August, I am ashamed to say that I cursed at my beloved colonel, which could have resulted in a court martial for me. In my defence, I was absolutely chin-strapped after setting off at 4 a.m. that morning and cycling for ten hours straight in 25 degrees heat.

The problems began when Vicky directed me to a campsite that didn't exist any more, even though it showed up on all her maps. The land near a place called Sublimity had recently been sold to a private dealer and although there were places for me to set up camp, the owner refused to let me stay there. When I told him, 'Look mate, I've just cycled a hundred kilometres to get here,' he reluctantly agreed, but insisted he would charge me $35 for an empty space with no amenities. 'And I'll only take cash,' he added unhelpfully.

I deliberately didn't carry much cash with me for fear of loss or theft and he refused to take my credit card, which meant I'd have had to cycle twenty-five miles into the nearby town of Albany, find a cash machine and pedal twenty-five miles back. I was beyond tired, so that wasn't an option. Vicky located a motel in Albany instead, which charged $55 for a room, bed, shower and breakfast.

'Everything worked out all right eventually but Chris was really pissed off with me,' she said. 'It was one of my worst mistakes and it came when he was at the far end.'

Dismissed!

To make it up to me she made sure I passed through a town called Dexter the following day, knowing that it would cheer me up. She was right. I stopped and filled my boots with photos of the Dexter Lake, Dexter United States Post Office, Dexter Market and Dexter Liquor. A quick Google search informed me that the town was named after the brand of Dexter stove that once sat in the postmaster's office in 1875. It was 'a good stove and so to be celebrated', I read. Unusual or uplifting places like that always made a crappy day bearable.

As a second consolation prize, Vicky booked me a much-needed rest stop at the Greenwaters Park bike trail campsite in Oakridge, in the foothills of the Cascade Range, with a beautiful river to swim in. Not far from my destination I rang Neil Deadman for a catch-up and it was great to hear his voice. He posted on Facebook later: 'Just received a phone call off Chris Graham. It was fantastic to hear from him as he was cycling through a forest in the middle of nowhere! He's doing really well and seems in great spirits. Every day is a challenge but he is definitely having more good days than bad. With the help of his partner Victoria who is almost as big a part of this journey as Chris himself. He would literally be lost without her!! Keep on pedalling brother. Proud of you and all you have achieved so far.'

After speaking to Neil and a good night's sleep, my faith in the world was restored and my energy levels refreshed. From inside my tent I gave my followers a 'grand tour', which I assured them wouldn't take long. In a few seconds I panned round to show my roll mat and sleeping bag plus my few valuables hanging up. I concluded, 'If in doubt – camp.'

From the moment I set off again, I became unreasonably obsessed about making it to the home of my old school friend Craig Calder in Long Beach, California, by Saturday 12 September. This meant I'd have to cover 820 miles in eleven days, averaging seventy-five miles a day. Based on my previous performance I knew I could probably manage it as my normal yomp was thirty miles in ninety minutes at a speed of between 10 and 20 mph, but only if the terrain and the weather were conducive. Pushing myself harder in California and parts of Nevada wouldn't allow me much rest, and the far bigger issue would be the heat.

The most direct route to Los Angeles would take me through Death Valley National Park, which meant cycling in daytime temperatures up to 41 degrees Celsius or 105 degrees Fahrenheit. Although I created my own breeze, which cooled me a little, I had to make sure that didn't give me a false sense of security and tempt me to push myself too much and oversweat. Appropriate re-hydration and rest stops could potentially become a matter of life and death.

People couldn't believe it when I told them what I intended to do. Death Valley is a zone of hazards and extremes – the lowest, driest and hottest region of North America. Its so-called 'points of interest' include Hell's Gate, Dante's View and Furnace Creek, the place where the highest tem-perature in the world was once recorded at 56.7 degrees Celsius or 135 degrees Fahrenheit.

Most drivers simply avoid this forbidding wil-derness during the warmest months because it's too hot for air conditioning: the radiators explode and cars can literally catch fire. Rental car com-panies refuse to hire vehicles to tourists there when it's very warm because of the number of breakdowns and cases of heat stroke amongst drivers. All along the road leading towards Death Valley, I found, there were warning signs listing the various precautions travellers should take. They advised people to inform someone of their exact route in case they went missing. They emphasised the importance of never underestimating how much water they'd need in the desert, and to carry a tarpaulin for cover. They warned that mobile phones might not work and that anyone crossing the desert should be equipped with maps and a GPS. They instructed drivers who broke down to stay with their vehicle as they'd be more easily visible for rescuers and could at least sit in its shade.

Looking down at Shirley, I sensed her slender shadow wouldn't do much to shade me from the ferocity of the midday sun, no matter how much Factor 50 sun cream I slathered on.

'You're crazy, man!' people told me. 'You'll die out there.'

'I'll be setting off at three a.m. and cycling mostly at night,' I countered.

'Don't you know how dangerous it is to travel anywhere in the desert at night?' they'd argue. 'You don't know what you might hit. What's the rush, anyway?'

'Manchester United are playing Liverpool in the derby,' I replied excitedly. 'I haven't seen my team play all season. Me and my mate Craig are going to watch it together on the telly.'

There were far too many times to mention during my journey when people stared at me as if I was stark staring mad, but the day I explained my urgency to cross one of the harshest known terrains on the planet just to watch a game of football, they clearly had me down as a lunatic.

What they didn't know was how good Craig had been to me and how much I was looking forward to seeing him. He and I grew up together in the Vale and went to Bollin Road Primary School together with Neil. We'd stayed in touch all these years and always had a few sherbets together whenever we were back home, or as Craig would say, we'd meet up for 'a sausage roll and a grin'.

He'd always been into cars and had worked for BMW in Altrincham as a teenager. He moved to the US with his parents when he was twenty-one, and turned his interest into a career. He now owns a successful company that buys vintage cars for clients from all over the world. Happily married to

Ofelia, with three kids, he was one of those who really helped me out when I was running out of money, and I'd never forget that. Watching Man U play with him was going to be on the highlights of my trip, especially if they won.

With that goal in mind, I crossed into California, known as 'The Golden State', headed for San Francisco where the wind came back to taunt me, chapping my lips and battering my face. At Vicky's insistence I stopped for a rest at Honey Lake, an extraordinary location near the Nevada border where in the searing heat the water had all but evaporated and there was nothing but sand. 'I tell you what, you could play a good game of football on that, couldn't you?' I joked. Man, it was hot, hot, hot out there.

A bit further on and flanked by the Sierra Nevada, I skirted Yosemite National Park, not far from where I'd been based with the military eleven years earlier and where we'd climbed Mount Whitney, which I could see in the distance. After months without rain, the area was tinder dry and forest fires became a fresh danger. I could smell the smoke and see the water planes flying in to bomb the flames with huge loads of water. I just hoped I didn't choke to death or inadvertently run into one of the wildfires and end up as barbecued Gurkha.

There were hardly any motels in the dry desert and campsites were few and far between at the small oases. Mirages formed by the shimmering heat haze deluded me into thinking there might be something or someone up ahead. Whenever I stopped to wild camp alone, I had to be especially vigilant when setting up my tent to make sure that I didn't have any freeloading houseguests such as scorpions, lizards, spiders or snakes. Good 'critter discipline' meant that I'd stamp everywhere first to scare them off and then zip everything up tight.

Vicks kept checking in on me every few hours, for which I was grateful. We both appreciated that Death Valley was an extremely dangerous place to be, especially when pushing myself to the limit. I was properly prepared, however, with plenty of water and food on board. Most of my cycling was done under cover of night, each of which was surprisingly sharp and had me piling on extra layers.

The big disadvantage about moving at speed in the dark was that I couldn't see snakes on the road, and I would accidentally ride over some of them with a sickening 'crump'. I doubt any of them would have survived 140 kg thumping over them, but they might well have whipped around to bite me before they expired. During the daytime, I could see the hazards – and there were plenty of rattlesnakes – so I gave them a wide berth wherever possible. The good news was that it was too hot for any airborne bugs.

The scariest and most worrying day was when I got food poisoning from a pastrami sandwich bought from a ramshackle shop, the only place for miles. Not long after wolfing it down, I started to be sick and then I threw up for two hours straight. Vicky was trying to get in touch with me and couldn't work out why I didn't respond, but I was spewing my guts up at the side of the road, leaving a few pavement pizzas for the rattlers to feast on.

I'd set off that morning at 4 a.m. and it was at least sixty miles to my next destination, so I was knackered.

When I eventually answered her calls and she heard how I was, she went into a blind panic to find me somewhere closer. By 11 a.m. it was getting incredibly hot, but there was nowhere to stop and I had no choice but to push on through 120 degrees. With my little Union flag valiantly fluttering away on Shirley, anyone passing us would surely have thought that only mad dogs and Englishmen go out in the midday sun. I eventually made it into the bed of my roadside motel that night several pounds lighter.

Amazingly, in that most inhospitable and inaccessible of landscapes, I was occasionally able to find a phone signal, which enabled me to post some video and photos online. The images did little to capture the wild beauty of the desert or the way the changing light hit the rocks. 'It's a bit like the Brecon Beacons, only bigger,' I said at one spot that was so windy the microphone could barely pick up my voice. 'I'm parched and I'm going to stop for a cup of tea,' I added.

My mate Craig commented, 'Are you sure you're cycling this? Never actually seen you ride. I bet you have a van hidden off camera.'

A few days later I reported that it had taken me three hours to climb to 4,000 feet in 122 degrees and only thirty minutes to freewheel down the other side. 'Lovely!' The day before I was due in Los Angeles I recorded a video that showed that according to my GPS it was already 96 degrees at 9 a.m. and that the wind was in my favour. 'These are the mountains,' I said, panning round to Deer Mountain and the rest of the spectacular range that fringed the desert, 'although I'm probably not doing them justice.' Citing my need to get there to watch a game of football, I signed off with 'Speak soon. Ciao!'

I made it to Craig's house in Long Beach with a day to spare. Best of all, Man United beat Liverpool 3-2. We watched it together at his house and then went to the Auld Dubliner Irish bar for a few wets. Then, for the next three days and nights, we hung out together windbagging and catching up. It was smashing to see Craig and we had a lot of fun, but the long-haired colonel was a bit worried about all my late nights and made me stay on an extra day just to get some rest.

'You know being tired is bad for your dementia,' she scolded. 'It's fine to have a couple of pints and a late night but staying up until two a.m. before you're about to start back to seventy miles a day is irresponsible, Chris. A rest day is a rest day and you need to be careful. You know this will catch up with you. You'll be tired and then you'll start feeling rough and that'll only make you more confused. It's a nightmare navigating you when you're like that!'

She was right, of course. She always was. I'd virtually given up drinking in the previous two years because I knew how much of an adverse effect it had on me. It had felt great to be normal for a few days, though, having fun with my mate. I'd enjoyed a few pints with Craig on the first night but after that I'd laid off it. What I had done was not get enough sleep, which meant that when I set off again on 21 September, I was still feeling somewhat the worse for wear. I could barely manage thirty miles a day and most of the music on my playlist seemed suddenly way too loud, especially bands like The Killers. In the end I settled on the gentle voice of Austin Cresswell, whose lyrics really touched a nerve. *Some day you will die but I'll be close behind you. I'll follow you into the dark...*

On 23 September, I was lying on my bed in my motel on the outskirts of Phoenix, Arizona, waiting for an oversized pepperoni pizza to be delivered. I'd had another bike fail that day with the front crank needing work, so I ended up hitching a lift into town to a bike shop to get a part, much to Vicky's distress. She worried when I hitchhiked, thinking I would be mugged or worse, but fortunately none of the people who stopped to pick me up turned out to be serial killers.

Not long after the deliveryman arrived, the phone rang and I heard Vicks squealing down the line. It took me a moment to remember that she was in London for the Just Giving awards ceremony. 'You only went and bloomin' well won!' she cried.

'What?'

'You won the prize for Best Endurance Fundraiser, soldier!'

'I don't believe it!' I cried.

'You'd better believe it, mate,' she said. 'If in doubt – win! I'm holding the award in my hand right now.'

'Bloody hell! Ha! Well, of course I knew I'd win all along.'

'You lie like a rug, Chris Graham!'

The date was 23 September. Although I'd just cycled several hundred miles across the San Bernardino Valley, through Palm Desert, and past the superheated Salton Sea before arriving in Phoenix, Arizona, she'd had a hell of a ride too. After three hours stuck in traffic with one of my old Army mates, Jason Garrett, at the wheel, she'd only made it to her seat at the London venue minutes before they announced the winner.

'It was a nightmare,' she said. 'The traffic was horrendous – nose to tail – and we were horribly late getting into town from Oxford. The people from Alzheimer's Research were calling and asking, "Where are you now?" Jason was really sick and almost throwing up en route. He kept winding the window down but he was determined not to miss it. We were so stressed.'

She was meant to be at the west London venue by 6.30 p.m., but at 7.45 she texted to tell them the satnav estimated they'd be there in fifteen minutes. 'Soon afterwards, I got yet another phone call telling me the show's organisers were about to run the videotape featuring Chris and I was panicking like mad. I told them I honestly didn't think we were going to make it in time and might even have to abandon the whole event. That's when they took a deep breath and said, "You have to get here NOW!" They had no choice but to ruin the surprise and blurt, "Chris is about to be announced as the winner!" I was staggered.'

They arranged a VIP parking place and had Vicky met by a man in a bowler hat who hurriedly escorted her into the venue. The actor Henry

173

Cavill was presenting another award as she walked in. Within two minutes, she was called up onto the stage to accept mine. She had hardly caught her breath and hadn't prepared a speech. Standing in front of hundreds of people with the TV cameras rolling she looked up, tried to ignore the celebrity table directly in front of her, and made up a speech as she went along.

'Wow!!' she began, still panting. Taking a breath, she said, 'Chris is currently about nine thousand miles into his journey and we have just realised that he isn't going to be home in April – he is in fact going to be home two weeks before Christmas and in time for our son's first birthday!'

She waited for the applause to die down before continuing on a more serious note. 'We have four children between us and three out of the four have a fifty per cent chance of inheriting the gene Chris carries and also succumbing to dementia at an early age. Alzheimer's Research is doing an amazing job and Chris and our family are so happy to do this, if nothing else to stop anyone else ever having to go through the trauma of watching a loved one go through it.'

Starting to get emotional, she added, 'I love Chris dearly and can't wait for him to get home.' She left the stage to rapturous applause with my elegant glass trophy gripped tightly in her hand.

That's my girl.

If in doubt – wing it.

10

'It is always our own self that we find
at the end of the journey.
The sooner we find that self, the better.'
ELLA MAILLART

Dementia Adventure Diary,
14 October 2015, Waco, Texas

Texas wasn't the place I'd thought it would be
with its rollercoaster roads and tumbleweed
brush. The landscape in the second largest state
after Alaska was mostly unremarkable, with
nothing much to see but oil wells and thousands
of wind turbines. More surprisingly, the weather
was so unpleasant that it made the riding extremely difficult.

Watching the television show *Dallas* in the
1980s had entirely shaped my perception of the
'Lone Star State'. Featuring the psychopathic oil
baron and cattle rancher J.R. Ewing from South-
fork Ranch, who once famously said, 'Blood is
thicker than water but oil is thicker than both,'
the programme depicted a high-rise cityscape
surrounded by miles of lush open ranchland full
of cows drenched in sunlight.

The part of Texas I traversed was barren by
comparison and there was hardly a head of cattle
to be seen. In a video I posted not long after I'd

crossed the state line, I said, 'I wasn't expecting to see JR because he's not around any more but I was expecting nice sunny weather. Instead, all it's done is rain, rain and rain, and the wind is shocking... I much prefer Manchester!'

After the 'Indian Territory' of Arizona, home of the Apaches, and then the 'Land of Enchantment' that is New Mexico, Texas seemed a bit dull by comparison. I'd just ridden through a stunning Wild West wilderness with jagged rock formations, pueblo towns, adobe houses, cacti, flora and fauna – plus a few tarantulas (fortunately only squashed ones on the road). The sunrises in the Wild West were especially marvellous and in an online sitrep I showed one as a thank you to all those who'd voted for me in the Just Giving Endurance Award.

'It was an honour to win,' I told them, 'I'm quite chuffed, to say the least.'

I must have been fired up because I went on to cycle more than seventy miles in a day not far from El Paso, an area that looked so much like a movie set that I half-expected Clint Eastwood to appear on his horse any minute to squint into the sun and tip his hat with an 'Adios, amigo.'

Home to cowhands and Stetsons, Texas may have seemed rather grey and flat, but it was full of super friendly people who were eager to help. And the food was fantastic – mostly ribs and steaks – and that suited me just fine, even if I felt like I needed a cowboy hat and some shit-kicking boots to fit in at some of the places I stopped to eat. At Lake Limestone Marina and Campground, the owners went the extra mile, giving me free bed and board once they found out what I was doing and why. They spoke to Vicks on the phone and cooed over Dexter, declaring, 'He's too cute!' I was set up like a king in one of their cabins on the lake and they even cooked me a huge tea of steak and mashed potato. Now that's what I call Texan hospitality.

I was grateful for another kind of hospitality a few days later when I got the shits from ingesting some bacteria in my CamelBak water carrier. Desperate for a place to stop where I wouldn't be seen from the road, I could hardly believe my luck when I came across a Portakabin toilet standing lone sentinel in the wilderness. It was undoubtedly meant for road workers and not foreign cyclists but – with my stomach churning – I dived in and proceeded to hog it for the next thirty minutes or more.

Whilst I was in there doing what I had to do (phoning Vicks and asking her to find me a motel – pronto), I was alarmed to hear a vehicle pull up outside. Peeping through a crack in the door in case someone had ungallant designs on my Shirley, I watched a burly rancher march up to the loo in cowboy boots with spurs. When I didn't emerge any time soon, he started hollering and banging on the door. There wasn't much I could do but sit it out and thankfully he finally buggered off, cross-legged.

The Texan countryside started to get a bit more interesting with rivers and trees further on as I rode through the unassuming city of Waco, not far from the site of the 1993 siege that took place after government officials raided the ranch of an armed religious sect. Seventy-six people died in a gun battle between the Branch Davidians and government officials and Waco will forever be associated with it.

I also rode through Davey Crockett National Forest, named after the legendary soldier, frontiersman and 'King of the Wild Frontier' who died fighting the Mexicans at the Alamo a few hundred miles south. Having been up close and personal with a few raccoons on my travels, I resisted the temptation to purchase a Davey Crockett hat complete with tail. Besides, where would I put it?

The shortest ride of my entire trip was in Texas, when I travelled a less than impressive sixteen miles in one day up a horribly deceptive incline somewhere near the small city of Cisco. I'd bitten off a big chunk of distance the previous day and had a long way to go the day after, so Vicky advised, 'Get that next hill out of the way then you can have a rest day.'

Several heavily laden lorries passed me as I climbed at about 1mph and the drivers tooted their horns with encouragement when they saw how much I was struggling. Then some US Army trucks overtook me and I got a few whistles and yells from their uniformed occupants. I was sweating like a kangaroo on trial by the time I made it to the top and couldn't help but grin when I saw that the soldiers had stopped, climbed out of their vehicle, and were waiting for me by the roadside to clap and cheer me on to the summit.

You made it, soldier!

Not long after that epic ride, my brakes seized again, so I had an unscheduled diversion north to 'historic' Nacogdoches, the oldest town in Texas, and a visit to the only bike shop for miles. As always, the staff were helpful and kind. As usual it was Vicks who helped me out, guided me in, told me when to rest and showed me where I could get something to eat and drink. She really is one in a million.

It was her birthday on 12 October, and I hoped to get to a motel somewhere with Wi-Fi that night in good time to be able to wish her happy birthday, face to face. Annoyingly, I had another brain fail and missed my turning, so by the time I found my way back to the correct route the sun had gone down and my only option was to camp. Riding along the road through a small town I rang Vicks and started singing 'Happy Birthday' at the top of my voice. A few minutes later I arrived at the campsite, which was in the middle of a forest. It was pitch black. Worse still, there were no lights and no member of staff to ask for a pitch, the Wi-Fi codes or even where I should dig in.

I figured I'd find somewhere and pay my way the next day, so I started looking for a place to pitch my tent in the dark. Vicks was still laughing at my antics in my earphones when I suddenly broke off as I stumbled across a middle-aged couple in the dark. I think I gave them a bit of a fright. 'Hiya,' I said, cheerfully, as Vicks listened in. 'Any idea where I can set up my tent?'

Despite the shock of bumping into a mad Brit apparently talking loudly to himself in the middle of a dark wood, those American campers were super friendly. 'My girlfriend's on the phone,' I explained, 'it's her birthday today.' Then I put her on speaker. Laughing, they said hello and wished her a happy birthday too.

The husband's name was Kevin and I found out later that he was a local politician. He took one look at my rig and said, 'That's a great looking set-up you have there. Where are you headed?' After I told him what I was doing and why, he and his wife kindly invited me into their RV for some delicious meat stew. Over a root beer after supper, we chewed the fat about politics and they asked me what I thought about everything from the British royal family to the UK's membership of Europe. When the subject moved to gun crime in the US, he spoke about the right to own a weapon and I said, 'I get that, but why do you need assault rifles?' And so the friendly but philosophical discussion went on well into the night.

It made a change for me to have a lively debate about life, the world and the universe, and – to his credit – my host didn't hold my conservative views against me. On the contrary, when it was time for bed he said, 'You may as well sleep in my hammock tonight.' He already had it rigged up next to his RV and knew it would save me setting up my tent in the dead of night. I accepted immediately. I love sleeping in hammocks and had originally taken one with me to North America, but it proved to be too heavy. In order to keep the weight down I'd ditched it along the way and given it to one of the lads to ship home.

That night in my free hammock, I slept like a fat bear cub. I set off early the next morning without a chance to say goodbye to my hosts, but the following day I saw that Kevin had friended me online and even posted something about me on his page: 'I will never forget meeting him,' he wrote. 'Pedal on, my new friend.'

Vicky never once grumbled about having to spend her birthday on her own without me. In fact, she never grumbled about anything much. There she was all alone back home, coping with me and two kids, work and her own private concerns about my health, our finances and our future. Even when she tripped coming down the stairs, breaking her toe and badly spraining her wrist, she just got on with it. That woman never failed to amaze me.

Meanwhile, I got on with what I had to do on the road. To break the monotony of the long roads that dipped and troughed for miles, I'd tune into my music and find myself a song that provided a beat to my rhythm, such as 'Billionaire' by Travie McCoy with Bruno Mars, or 'Payphone' by Maroon 5. To ease my aches and pains, I'd try to vary my position slightly in the saddle, standing on the pedals while freewheeling, sitting upright or resting heavily on the handlebars – anything to keep up the willpower to carry on pedalling. Someone sent me a poster that said *Eat. Sleep. Bike. Repeat,* which summed up my daily routine precisely. I loved it so much I posted it online.

As I left the warm hospitality of Texas and crossed into the 'Pelican State' of Louisiana (which indeed has great flocks of pelicans), I was making such good progress that I felt as if I could start to see the light at the end of the tunnel.

Vicky felt the same way and on 14 October, two days after her birthday, she felt confident enough to book my flight home. In a series of phone calls

181

she even managed to persuade Iceland Air to waive the £1,000 levy I should have incurred for flying on Christmas Eve. When a kind lady manager rang to tell her what the airline had agreed, Vicky burst into tears with gratitude. Bless Iceland Air's woolly Nordic socks.

Beyond excited, Vicky couldn't wait to announce the news online: 'Coming Home! Update from Mission Control: Flight home is now booked! ETA 11.30am 24 December.' We were immediately inundated with congratulations and good luck messages, with friends calling me a 'true Manc' and saying how pleased they were that I'd be back in time for Christmas.

Not wishing to push my luck, I advised caution and replied, 'Hi all, it's not in the bag yet. However as long as I keep up the same daily distances I should be okay. We cannot second-guess Mother Nature. Fingers crossed the weather will be kind to me.'

Despite my public scepticism, I was quietly confident I could get back in time for Dexter's first Christmas, and the second for Vicky and me. I was certainly determined to try. It wasn't just about completing my ride any more, or even about how we'd continue to fund everything, it was about getting home and being with Vicks and our beautiful baby boy, both of whom I missed with a yearning ache that couldn't be eased.

One of our best songs, and perhaps the most poignant of all on my playlist – it made me well up each time it came around – was the Rihanna song with the line, *We found love in a hopeless place*. And it's true – we did.

I never thought I stood a monkey's chance with Vicky when I met her properly on Saturday 15 February 2014 at Andy Harrison's leaving party, at a military social centre near Brize Norton. Andy – H – is the bloke I've known since Chepstow and the one who used to call out, 'Slow down, Gurkhs!' on runs out of Abingdon. Coincidentally, he was dating Jenny, one of Vicky's oldest friends, whose father had served alongside hers in bomb disposal. Jenny invited us both to H's surprise do, not realising that we'd already met many years earlier at that pub in Abingdon when I was just eighteen. Neither of us remembered that day, but we both knew we fancied each other from the start.

Vicks claims I was drunk that night (what a slur on my character!) and says that when I sidled over to her near the dance floor with what may be the worst chat-up line ever – 'Nice teeth!' – she either didn't hear or didn't understand me. Instead, she walked off to dance with her daughter Katy, who'd just celebrated her tenth birthday. Undaunted, I repeated my line to Vicky at the bar later while she was chatting to H, who – I discovered afterwards – was telling her what a top bloke Gurkhs was.

Her response to my comment about her outstanding dentistry wasn't quite what I hoped. Staring at me as if I was bonkers, she replied, 'What am I supposed to say to that?' Although she was smiling, I could tell that she was playing it as cool as the Fonz and pretending not to be beguiled by my irresistible charms. What I didn't know was that, at thirty-nine and single, she had been on her own with Katy for almost a decade and had no intention of bringing a man into their lives unless she was one hundred and fifty per cent certain that he was a keeper.

No one can ever claim that this soldier isn't a trier, so I launched into my second best chat-up routine – wiggling my sticky-out ears and flaring my nostrils. At least that elicited a laugh, and what a pretty laugh it was. She said later that it was like watching some sort of crazy mating dance, and, yes, I was dancing around her and flirting with her and doing my utmost to keep her attention focused on me for the rest of that night. I was due to stay at a friend's house in Cirencester but when I saw Vicks leaving with H, Jenny and his family to get a taxi home from their house, I blew off my mate and joined them instead.

Uninvited, I walked home with H, pretending to be cool myself as I chatted to him a few paces behind Vicky and Jen. When her taxi arrived to take her and Katy home, I walked the thirty yards to the main road with her until she turned and asked me where I thought I was going. 'Home with you!' I replied, with a grin.

Laughing, she told me, 'Oh, no you're not!' Having suggested that I bugger off, she got on her way, but not before she'd given me the means to contact her via Facebook. An hour or so later and with my head still spinning as I was crashed out, I sent her the following message: *Hey Vicky, I hope you're well. At the mo I'm lying on the settee in H's house. I'm wide awake and bored. It was great meeting you tonight. I'm an honest lad and yes I do fancy you. It would be nice to meet you again. Speak soon hun xxx.*

184

She didn't see my message until later the next day, and only after she'd turned up at the house all dolled up did she discover that I'd already left. 'I was gutted,' she said. 'I thought Chris was really fit and good-looking and I feared that, once sober, he wouldn't look twice at me. There was something special about him and it wasn't just the sob story H had told me about him being in a children's home or badly burned as a kid. He had real charisma.'

Having missed me by minutes, she messaged me back: *It was lovely to meet you too. I'm ever so flattered you fancy me. The feeling is mutual. Sorry we didn't get much time to chat. I felt awkward with my daughter being there. Be good to meet up without distraction. I am a shy one when it comes to guys but I'm an honest lass too. Hope your hangover isn't too bad – speak soon.* Tellingly, both of us saved those messages and have them on our phones to this day.

Vicks said later that the more she thought about me, the more she knew that I was something special. 'It was Fate from the minute we met. The magnetism was there and there was no getting away from it. There was nothing on this planet that would have prevented us from being together.'

I couldn't get her out of my head either, so when I rang her later that day I decided to be straight and tell her everything up front. First, though, I sat on my own for a long time staring at my phone in my hand, trying to think of the best way to say it. How do you break it to someone you've only just met that you're going to die in a few years?

My sister Lizzie had exactly the same dilemma the previous year when she met her boyfriend

185

Kevin after her marriage ended. Like me, she wanted to be honest with him from the start. In the end, she just went for it and Kev was great. It was he who encouraged her to finally have the test. She and Angie went ahead at the same time and, thankfully, both tested negative. They didn't have the 'daft gene' after all, which meant that their children had no chance of inheriting it. I was absolutely made up for them.

'So, you're just daft then?' I told Lizzie, joking about it as always, even though we both knew my situation was far from funny.

Get on with it, Gurkha.

'I really like you,' I finally blurted to Vicky on the telephone once I'd plucked up the courage. 'But there's something you should know. I've got a rare genetic disorder that's likely to give me early dementia. My brother has it but my two sisters don't. The chances are I'll die sooner than most, although I still think I'm going to beat it or they'll find a cure in time.'

There was a long silence down the end of the line, so I added, 'Oh, and I'm going to cycle around North America later this year to raise money for Alzheimer's Research and the ABF. You can come out and do a leg of it with me if you like!'

I could sense her shock but, to my surprise, I heard her say, 'That's fine by me.'

'Really?' I asked, hardly believing what I was hearing. 'I'm talking about Alzheimer's.'

'And?' she replied. 'I know what it is, Chris. A good friend of my mum works with the elderly. I had a Saturday job serving tea and biscuits in the nursing home she ran. My ex's mother has Alz-heimer's so I'm accustomed to the fall-out from dementia on a family. When do you want to meet up?'

What she didn't tell me was that she wasn't a stranger to inherited medical problems either. There was a history of heart attacks in her own family, with her grandfather, uncle and father all having them unusually young. Needless to say, as soon as our telephone conversation ended she quickly looked up my gene to see what it meant, a step that started her on a lifelong quest into research about my condition.

'All he told me at the beginning was that he was having loads of tests because he'd been found to have the gene,' she said. 'Neither of us really knew what it would mean, but he seemed unaffected to me and was very hopeful of a cure. In spite of my bravado, I was secretly very torn and I knew I had Katy to consider as well. I simultaneously wanted to run towards Chris and run away from him, if that makes sense. What helped me to stay, though, was that I'd never met anyone so courageous or someone with such a glass half full attitude to life. That was the man I was about to fall head over heels in love with.'

We spoke every day for the next three weeks, and then on 7 March she invited me to stay at her home near Brize Norton while Katy was away with her father. When Vicks picked me up from Oxford train station she was so nervous she was shaking (I have that effect on women). We were meant to be going out for dinner that night but we never made it out of the house and stayed

187

there for the next nine days. We did manage to get up and out once or twice and our first official date was at the Chequers pub in Brize Norton, where we had supper with H and Jenny. I guess we got under each other's skin right from the start.

Vicky's friends and family were very protective of her and understandably cautious about me, especially being a squaddie, but her mother Lynn decided to reserve judgement until she met me. Fortunately, I won her over too and we've been best friends ever since. Lynn had been in the Army too until she became a mum, social worker and full-time carer. She was in logistics for the Women's Royal Army Corps or WRAC as a young woman and was separated from Vicky's dad John, but had then married Ken, a flight mechanic with the United States Air Force. She knew all about life and death, what it was like in the military, and how those in the services often had a stronger sense of seizing the moment.

As Vicks told her, 'I can't walk away from Chris, Mum, because if I do I'll be walking away from the best thing that ever happened to me.'

By that time she and I were too crazy about each other to worry about anything other than working out how we could be together. Those initial few weeks were magical and gave me the first major boost I'd had in a while, because ever since my second marriage ended in Nepal in early 2013, my life had taken a series of unexpected and unwelcome turns.

My nightmare began the day I decided to do the right thing and inform those in command that I had a medical condition that could ultimately affect my performance as a soldier. I was still flying high at the time and had no serious or obvious symptoms. Yes, I was a bit forgetful and didn't always feel fully on top of things in my head, but my work didn't seem to suffer and not one person remarked on it, so no alarm bells were ringing. I'd already adopted a few coping strategies and masking tactics to help myself, including writing everything down and memorising the things I needed to be really clear about.

I'd also been reassured about the progress of dementia in our family on a recent trip home when I'd spent some time with my brother Tony. Although easily confused and physically weak, he was doing better than I'd imagined and had even been well enough for me to take him to see United and Everton play at Old Trafford. I hoped that by staying fit and keeping myself in peak condition, I'd delay the inevitable for even longer. I was challenging my brain constantly and had just passed my maths GCSE (albeit by the skin of my teeth on a weasel of a course) as part of my bid for promotion to warrant officer, 2nd class. I was due to take an English exam too, which would have been hard for someone who struggles with Mancunian let alone English, but I know I'd have managed it.

Reassuringly, I was promoted anyway. And the news came to me in a very unconventional way and in a very unusual location. It was June 2013 and I was doing some adventure training and leadership skills in the Himalayas with half a dozen fellow soldiers. We were tasked to climb two major peaks in three weeks. Near the summit of a mountain called Imja Tse, also known as Island Peak, my chief of staff suddenly found a spot where he could pick up a phone signal and took a call from our colonel.

When they'd finished speaking, he turned to me in front of everyone else and said, 'Congratulations Staff Graham, you've got your promotion to WO2. At six thousand metres, that must be one of the highest promotions anyone has ever received!'

My mates crowded around me to pat me on the back and cry, 'Well done, Gurkhs!'

I was made up, and I knew that being a warrant officer would take me neatly to the end of my mandatory twenty-four years' service in January 2015, with retirement on a full military pension. Historically, the Ministry of Defence refuses to take into account the two years soldiers like me spend in the junior leaders in its calculations of military pensions, despite widespread calls to recognise what is known as 'boy service'. We in the Army refer to it as 'the extra two we did for the Queen'. Still, beggars can't be choosers.

It hardly seemed possible that almost a quarter of a century had passed since I'd taken the bus from the children's home and turned up wet behind the ears at the Army Careers Office in central Manchester asking to sign up. I'd seen and done so much since that day when I was sweet sixteen, and I wouldn't have changed a single moment of it.

Given the choice, I'd have stayed in the military for ever because I loved it so much. There were a few options for people to stay on sometimes, but the government had recently announced massive cuts in the defence budget, including a reduction of personnel from 102,000 to 80,000. So I knew I wouldn't have a choice.

My final posting had already been decided – it would be to the British Army garrison at Paderborn in Germany, which was about to be merged with another at Gutersloh and become a 'super garrison' called Westfalen, home of the 20th Armoured Brigade. Being there would be a very different environment from the gentle pace I'd enjoyed at the post office in Nepal working with the Gurkha recruitment team. It would also mean a return to handling a gun. After a break of two years I'd need to undertake a weapons handling test on a range, something that required me to be of sound mind.

Even though I knew I could dismantle and reassemble a weapon blindfolded, I realised that if I didn't tell my commanding officers about my dementia and accidentally had an ND – a negligent discharge – then that would be a chargeable offence of 'culpable carelessness' and would undoubtedly be the end of the Army for me. It was this thought which finally made me decide to pay a visit to the regimental doctor in Kathmandu.

'I've come to tell you that I've been diagnosed with a rare gene that can bring on early dementia, sir,' I told him. 'It hasn't activated yet but the tests show that I have the same thing that killed my father and is affecting other members of my family. I thought it best to inform you before Germany.'

He took some notes and told me that he was

now obliged to notify HQ. Nodding my under-standing, I saluted and left, hoping that would be the end of it. Little did I know. From that moment on, my career prospects imploded with a 'boom'. Within weeks I was put on light duties. My posting to Paderborn was cancelled and I was told that when my tour finished in early October I'd be sent to South Cerney instead. My friends in Nepal gave me a fantastic send-off and I promised I'd see them on the flip side. It had been a great tour and I'd seen and done so many fascinating things that I was very sad to be leaving.

I had a few days at home to acclimatise to life in Blighty and it was fantastic to be back with my friends and family. 'Football and music mad, friendly and down-to-earth citizens. Manchester rocks!' I posted online from my new forward base camp – Neil Deadman's sofa. I was also very happy to be going back to Cerney because I had loads of mates there, including Pete Davies, but there was no chance for a big reunion as I was only there for one day. My orders on arrival were to report to the Catterick Garrison and appear before a medical board. Taking Neil with me for moral support, I took my seat in front of a three-member panel who appeared to be extremely concerned, which made me all the more sur-prised to hear them tell me that my promotion was indefinitely on hold until the medical staff had been able to fully assess me.

Perhaps I was being naïve, but I hadn't expected that at all. I'd made the grade, after all, and noth-ing had changed as far as I was concerned. No matter what role they found for me next, I could surely still carry it out as a WO2? More worryingly for my future, unless I gained my promotion I wouldn't leave the service with the higher level of pension I'd been working towards and had already unofficially achieved. There was no time to quiz them, though, as my next orders were to report immediately to the Defence Medical Rehabilitation Centre at Headley Court in Epsom, Surrey.

Headley Court is a huge Victorian mansion set in eighty acres. It's the place where all injured British military personnel are sent for rehabilitation, and it has a hydrotherapy pool, gym, nurses, prosthetic specialists and the most incredible rehab facilities. For me, it was a bit like being back in the children's home though, as I had to share a dorm with four other soldiers with various physical or mental disabilities. I felt completely out of place and something of a fraud amongst the limbless or those who were suffering from severe post-traumatic stress disorder.

The whole place had the feel of a military hospital. We were still classed as working soldiers but didn't have to wear uniforms, just sports kit. Under the supervision of doctors, military case workers, civilian social workers and medical orderlies I underwent a battery of tests and was sent off to classes in everything from cooking to horse riding, swimming, tennis, running, cognitive and physical therapy. I soon made friends among the crew, some of whom jovially dubbed me 'the Memory King'.

Although I had a good laugh with some of those crazy cats, it wasn't much fun being stuck at Headley. I had to undergo test after test and felt sometimes as if I was being treated like a child. There was art therapy and play therapy and I was asked an untold number of questions about how I was feeling, what I could remember, what I planned to do once I left the Army. When I told them that I wanted to do a charity bike ride in my final 'resettlement' year, they seemed to approve and switched some of my activities to those more suited to my ongoing fitness regime.

In fact, the medical and military personnel at Headley were so enthusiastic about my plan that I began to hope they would help me come up with a scheme to organise it. My expectation was that I'd be doing the ride with Army sponsorship while raising money for the ABF and Alzheimer's Research and could start it sooner rather than later in order to complete it before the end of my service. One thing they appeared to be worried about was that even though my mate Neil was still planning to ride alongside me at that point, we'd be doing it unsupported. They advised me to have back-up, with a proper support vehicle, but I wasn't keen on the idea. Mark Beaumont had done it all by himself with a handheld video camera, after all.

I was still in Headley Court with my future undecided when I met Vicky in early 2014, which was one of the reasons I had to get the early train back to Surrey after H's party. Two weeks after meeting her, on 27 February, I was discharged from the rehab unit and told to wait at home until further notice on a type of gardening leave. That wasn't what I wanted to hear and all this waiting was killing me.

194

A few of my comrades in arms from Headley posted some nice comments online and wished me well. 'Good luck, buddy,' wrote one. 'Enjoy the freedom and try not to forget us too quickly.' Another wrote, 'Best of luck Chris and please keep us posted as we like to know how you're doing.'

Having told the Army that I'd be staying in Manchester with my mate Neil or on the sofa at my sister Lizzie's, they made arrangements for me to come under the supervision of the Personnel Recovery Unit in Preston. This involved reporting to an officer regularly and undertaking periodic week-long 'enrichment activities' that included rock climbing, skiing, sailing and running, as well as ongoing medical and psychological tests. I was still a soldier on duty, just not deployable, one officer told me.

I felt like a hamster on a wheel.

I'd decided to visit other friends and a few of my shipmates working abroad that year, but once I fell for Vicks, I applied to be supervised by a closer PRU at Aldershot in Surrey, a place I knew well from my earliest days in the Army. The other great thing about staying at her place just a few miles away from RAF Brize Norton was that I could have all my medicals there, so the military approved my move. The doctors at Brize were then tasked with collating the results of my tests at Headley, as well as liaising with the team from the Dementia Research Unit in London. Then they could decide my prognosis before a decision on my future was made. I was informed that the results would be reported to me later in the summer, when I hoped to receive news of my final posting.

Although I was itching to get back to soldiering as soon as possible, I loved spending some quality time with Vicks, who threw herself into helping me plan my charity bike ride. With the clock ticking, I was even more eager to get going. By the time I received a letter in the post summoning me to appear before a medical board to hear my results on 3 June, I was relieved to finally have a date.

'At last!' I exclaimed. 'Now we can hear the decision and get on with it.' Vicks and I figured that Neil and I still had enough time left to start the ride that year. I couldn't wait to get started.

If in doubt – crack on.

11

'Difficult roads often lead to beautiful destinations.'

UNKNOWN

Dementia Adventure Diary, 26 October 2015, Lakeland, Florida

My ride across Louisiana and Alabama, on my way to Florida and the most southerly point of my ride, was probably the most relaxing of my entire trip. It took me only five days to travel five hundred miles, the weather was balmy, the wind was behind me and a lot of the countryside reminded me of England.

Since the day I'd first discovered that I had the daft gene I'd set myself a bucket list of things to do and places to see before I became unable to. Although I'd been to the Carolinas on exercises before, I'd always wanted to see this part of the United States and it didn't disappoint. The sunrises over the Gulf of Mexico were especially beautiful and I stopped to watch them with the same sense of wonder I'd had since I was a kid camping out in the Bollin Woods.

Psychologically, it also felt good to be approaching the third of my four corners of that great continent after exactly six months on the road. From Key Largo I'd be on the home straight and pushing north with a three-day rendezvous a month later with my mate Pete Davies in Washington DC, before setting off again on my final five-hundred-mile push.

Southern hospitality is legendary and everyone I met was very friendly, with those charming accents that could allow them get away with almost anything, even the repeated assumption that I was an Australian. I rode through places like Eunice and Baton Rouge, passed north of New Orleans and through a town called Biloxi in Mississippi, the 'Magnolia State'. I cycled south of Mobile, Alabama, keeping an eye out for the pretty yellowhammer birds that the state was named after, before heading for the border near Pensacola in Florida, the 'Sunshine State'.

I enjoyed some delicious Southern cooking, including fried chicken and tomato pie, country ham, collard greens and cornbread. I never tried the grits (an unappetising-looking dish), but I loved the high-calorie hush puppies (a kind of savoury batter ball), and peach cobblers washed down with a glass of iced tea.

Even the road kill was different in the South, with dead porcupines and armadillos as common a sight as we might see pheasants or hedgehogs. I had to be careful not to hit any of the bloated corpses in my way as they might well have thrown me off my bike, especially in the dark. Worse still, I tried to avoid the slippery remnants of the carcasses that had quite literally exploded in the heat.

For a day or two I rode right alongside the coast at the Gulf Islands National Seashore, and that was especially stunning. Vicks found me a cycle path that took me past some exquisite houses right by the Gulf. It was a very peaceful part of my ride with its bleached white beaches, sand dunes, reed beds and shimmering flocks of sea-birds. The air was warm and there was a gentle sea breeze. Each time I stopped at a campsite or roadside diner to enjoy some delicious seafood, there was great music to listen to as well – a warm mix of Cajun and country which seemed to be playing all the time and soon had people singing or strumming along.

In Tallahassee, I stayed overnight with Vicks's cousin Ashley and her husband Kevin. Vicky's aunt Jean had moved out to America with her husband years ago after meeting him at a USAF base in the UK. Ashley was born there. Jean, who is originally from Sunderland, made me a cottage pie and brought it over for my tea, and it was a lovely reminder of home cooking. I'd never met any of them before and the last time Vicky saw Ashley she was a toddler, but once she contacted them they immediately opened their house and their hearts to me before sending me on my journey.

Once again, I was reminded of the innate goodness of all those who went out of their way to help me. Not just friends and family, but complete strangers who immediately identified with my plight and fully supported what I was trying to achieve. I was staggered to hear how many of those I met were affected by dementia in some form or other. Everyone seemed to have had parents or partners, siblings or friends stricken with it and to be struggling with the consequences.

The World Health Organisation identifies dementia as a public health priority that requires coordinated global action. It estimates that currently worldwide there are 47.5 million people with dementia, plus 7.7 million new cases every year. There are 850,000 people living with dementia in the UK alone, and their care costs at least £26 billion every year. By 2030, it is predicted, there will be 75.6 million sufferers worldwide, a figure which will rise to 135.5 million by 2050. By the middle of the century two people will develop the disease every minute.

Alzheimer's is the most common cause of dementia and contributes to at least sixty per cent of cases, the vast majority of whom are over sixty. Known as 'the silent disease', it is generally assumed that it only robs people of their mental capacity when they are old, but that is far from the truth. There are more than 42,000 sufferers in the

UK alone aged between thirty-five and sixty-five, victims of early-onset or 'young onset' dementia like me, although the numbers with a rare genetic defect like ours are only in their hundreds.

The cruel deterioration of cognitive function is believed to be caused by the build-up of the abnormal protein known as amyloid, which surrounds the brain cells in sticky masses and destroys the chemical connections between them so that they start to shrink rapidly. Once this shrinkage begins, it becomes a death sentence for those who have it and a life sentence for their carers, friends and families. The brain of someone with Alzheimer's will end up developing holes until it looks like Swiss cheese and, at death, will be about a third of the size of a healthy brain.

My brother Tony was a classic example. As his mental impairment worsened and he incrementally lost his job, his ability to drive, to walk and talk properly, so his world became smaller and smaller. By the time I set off on my Dementia Adventure, he was bedridden and only able to express himself through his smiles. Two weeks before I turned my first pedal in Canada, his family posted something on his public Facebook page that he had written while he still could. They never posted anything again.

Like any disease it has a cause, it has a progression, and it could have a cure. My greatest wish is that my children, our children, the next generation, do not have to face what I am facing. But for the time being I'm still alive. I know I'm alive. I have people I love dearly. I still have moments in the day of pure happiness and joy. And please do not think that I am suffering. I am not suffering. I am struggling. Struggling to be a part of things. To stay connected to who I once was. So live in the moment I tell myself. It's really all I can do. Live in the moment.

In the previous year he'd suffered seizures and then the symptoms of a stroke that affected his right side, especially his arm, and began to render him incontinent. When things got too difficult at home, he was placed in an assessment unit and then on a mental health ward. For a brief time he went into assisted housing and was doing well, but then he had a fall after another possible seizure and banged his head. He ended up unconscious in a hospital geriatric ward where he almost died after medical staff instructed he be given 'nil by mouth', leaving him to dehydrate and almost starve. As soon as his family went to visit him, they were horrified. After making an official complaint they arranged for him to be moved to another ward, but a doctor there told them bluntly, 'He has Alzheimer's. All we are doing is delaying the inevitable.'

Tony is a fighter – like me, like Mum and Dad, Angie and Lizzie. He grew up in the Vale, after all, and he wasn't ready to give up yet. He nearly didn't make it and remained in hospital for five months, but eventually he was well enough to be moved to a private nursing home in Timperley, near Altrincham, where he remains today having round-the-clock care – the youngest patient in a home full of the elderly. Terribly weak and with severe muscle wastage, however, he never bounced back from his fall and his quality of life changed completely.

Visiting him became harder for us all. Jayne and their sons went as often as they could and Jan still travelled from Wales every week to see him. Lizzie was a frequent visitor too but I didn't go as much as I should, perhaps because it felt as if each time I did I was staring at my own future. Whenever I did make the effort I'd lark around, ever the cheeky chappie trying to raise a laugh, but I found it heartbreaking that Tony couldn't interact, or even tell me to bugger off like he used to. I think he knew it was me from the way he smiled but he couldn't communicate in any meaningful way. Seeing him like that, or even thinking about him, is the one thing that can reduce me to tears.

In 2015, Jayne came across something in her son's schoolwork that also made me weep. For a project entitled 'Simply the Best,' Richard nominated me. He wrote that although I was in the Army and never saw my family much, 'He's the funniest guy I know... He helps when I'm sad ... and life's a bit against me. When I think of him, everything's better.' He went on to say that I was always there for him and his family. Bless his heart.

As Tony's condition worsened, his family agreed to have him listed as 'DNR' – Do Not Resuscitate – but that would only end his suffering if he had a heart attack or developed some other life-threatening condition, or caught pneumonia. Otherwise, he'd just continue the way he was. I found it pitiful to see my big brother like that. We wouldn't let an animal suffer in the same way. If I'd had a gun I could have put him out of his misery, but I wasn't allowed to – and nor was anyone else. If there was the chance of a cure in time then maybe it would have been more bearable, but there wasn't and it was no life being in bed all day, fed through a tube, turned by nurses and having his bum wiped. In spite of my upbeat behaviour in his company, secretly I couldn't wait to get away.

The knowledge that Tony's fate would be mine, and the fear that it might be the same for his boys, as well as for my children (who were still all too young to be tested), weighed heavily on my mind. Not long after I was first diagnosed, my ex-wife Kimmy broke the news to Natalie and Marcus that I had the mutant gene, as well as making the shocking revelation that they had a chance of inheriting it too. At the age of nine and ten, they were understandably confused and upset.

My next conversation with them on Skype was extremely hard. 'What your mum has said is true,' I admitted, before trying to brush it off. 'But I'm fine – and remember, you have just as much chance of *not* having the gene as you do of having it. You could be knocked down by a bus any day, so try not to dwell on it. Besides, by the time you're as ancient as me, dementia probably won't even exist any more.'

On the one or two occasions that I saw my kids each year, I made sure to be on top form and prove to them that their dad was just fine and dandy, so that they had nothing to worry about – yet. Probably because they were afraid of the answer, they never even asked me about it. Once they became teenagers, they began to ask Vicks a few questions about how I was or comment on the fact that I seemed more forgetful, but they never said anything to me. I guess history was repeating itself when it came to not discussing things in our family. It made me appreciate for the first time how difficult it must have been for Mum to talk about it with us kids – if she ever even fully appreciated that the condition ran through Dad's side of the family. I now know that it's far easier to bury your head in the sand.

There would be no head burying for me, though, because in June 2014, I was due to face the Army medical board at Aldershot and discover my fate. Although everyone at Headley Court had treated me very well for the four months that I'd been there, it had been unsettling to have my competence constantly challenged and I began to wonder what they had in mind for me next. As long as they let me soldier on until then in some way, I'd be happy. I speculated on all the different jobs I could do, especially after I'd seen so many severely disabled men and women take on useful roles despite serious physical injury. If a one-armed soldier could operate a field telephone or an airman with no legs could type up reports, then I could be of service too. I was able-bodied and could easily work in a sorting office, run a mess, man an Army recruitment office, or – better still – become a physical fitness trainer for young recruits. I chuckled when I imagined them pleading, 'Slow down, Gurkha!'

All ex-service personnel are allowed several months in their final year of service to prepare them for civilian life, what we call Civvy Street. We are offered leave, support and training as well as resettlement grants for the first three years and 'career transition' advice. If you have a nice CO – commanding officer – and have had a good career in the military then you can usually count on six months with full pay to do what you like, while the other six months are spent preparing yourself for the massive upheaval of a life out of uniform.

On the rare occasions I ever thought about my long-term future – and aside from the madcap schemes I had with Neil Deadman to one day run a burger van or own a chippy – I'd imagined I'd apply for a job at the Post Office, but the charity bike ride was always going to come first. My dream was to take my lump sum, get on my bike and go.

The prospect of the Aldershot medical board and the worry about what they might say was making me increasingly nervous but I was determined to remain optimistic, especially since I had Vicks by my side. I'd virtually moved in with her by then, although she claimed I was 'taking over' when I emptied half of her wardrobe (including her old maternity dresses) to accommodate my kit. Then I threw a bespoke quilt some kind grandmothers at Headley Court had made for me across her bed.

'My bed has been Gurkha-fied,' she wrote on social media with a photo of said quilt emblazoned with my name and the insignia of the Commandos. 'Apparently military style is in vogue. Just waiting for matching curtains and trip wires!'

Guilty as charged.

What she didn't mind so much was me taking

her out and buying her some new clothes. I'd never met a woman before who spent so little on herself and I wanted to spoil her.

Then at 4 p.m. on 2 June, the day before I was due to appear before the men in white coats and hear what the Army had in mind, Vicky came home from work looking dreadful. She held down a number of jobs, but that day she'd been caring for a friend with multiple sclerosis and I wondered if it had been a difficult few hours for her. I was in the kitchen brewing up a wet when she walked in and made an announcement that changed everything.

'I'm pregnant.' Her face was white and I noticed that she was shaking and had been crying.

'You what?' I replied, stunned.

'You heard me.'

'What? How? Fuck! What are we going to do?'

She burst into tears and we started arguing, and I honestly didn't know what to say. It was only later that I learned that she'd suspected for a few days and had stopped at a supermarket on her way to work that morning to buy a pregnancy testing kit. She took it into the toilet and when she saw that it was positive she sat shaking in the cubicle, terrified of the consequences.

'I really didn't want to go home and tell Chris,' she said later. 'I knew it wasn't what either of us wanted. We had only just met, we were taking precautions, and although we loved each other I knew that we were still in the first flush and that this could destroy us. From the moment I told him, he looked like a rabbit in the headlights and kept saying that he didn't want to father another

child that might inherit what he had. I understood but I was bawling my eyes out. In the end
I went for a long walk on my own because I
couldn't bear to see the sadness and worry in his
face.'

The news was far too much to take in for both
of us, especially with the medical board coming
up the following morning. Plus Vicky's young
daughter Katy had just come home from school
and we didn't want her to overhear our conversation. In the end we went to bed early and tried
to file the information away until we knew what
was going to happen with me in the Army.

As we drove grey-faced to Aldershot early the
next morning I realised that everything hung in
the balance. Quite apart from the fact that any
future child of mine had a 50/50 chance of inheriting the gene, my career was on the line, and I was
planning to bugger off on a year-long charity bike
ride any day, which would hardly be fair to Vicky
or the baby. All we could do was go ahead and find
out what the military had decided, see where
they'd send me next, and take it from there.

The medical board was held in an airless office
in a bland building and can't have lasted more
than thirty minutes. Vicky, who hadn't slept and
was already suffering from morning sickness,
filed in next to me like a shadow and we sat at a
desk facing three doctors in uniform. My case-
worker, an Army captain, took a seat at the back
of the room. The person who did all the talking
was a female medical officer who began by telling
us how all the various test results were devised
and how carefully they'd been evaluated, checked

and rechecked. As she droned on, leading up to something, Vicks and I both started to get a horrible sinking feeling in our stomachs.

Finally she said something to the effect of 'The results show that you have severe cognitive impairment, Staff Graham. You probably only have another seven good years left.' She added that the tests proved I was no longer capable of handling a weapon, when the first rule of soldiering is that you must be able to handle a weapon. 'You are no longer fit for that purpose,' she concluded. 'You cannot therefore remain in the military.'

I sat bolt upright and sensed Vicky's body stiffen too, before she slumped back in her chair. She told me later that she didn't know whether to puke or pee. There had been little attempt to soften the blow. The officer just blurted out what nobody else had ever told us to that point – that I'd probably be dead of dementia within seven years. Even the captain at the back of the room gave a sharp intake of breath.

As Vicks and I both struggled to take the information in, I heard the board spokeswoman add that although I'd hoped to complete the charity bike ride as part of my final year, because I was planning to do it unsupported the Army couldn't insure me and in this instance they wouldn't be able to allow it. Barely pausing for breath, she added with something approaching a smile, 'You can do it once you're out, though ... whilst you can.'

I was so shocked I couldn't even speak at first. There was too much bad news to digest. I'd truly thought that the Army would let me wear my boots right until the end. Instead, by the time I'd gone through resettlement and the various processes required by the regulations, they'd be kicking me out just six months short of my twenty-four years' service and without my warrant officer's pension. That would mean a much-reduced lump sum and a medical discharge. Never for one moment did I think that the Army I adored wouldn't take care of me to my last day of service. I was gutted.

I didn't cry, although I felt close to it. Still reeling, I think I finally managed to say 'Really?' or something similar, to which the reply was that there was no comeback from this. I would not be allowed to appeal the medical board's decision, only the employment decision. Stunned, I looked across at Vicky, who seemed close to collapse.

Dazed, she let me lead her out of that horrible room and then she clung to me silently, completely unable to summon up any words of comfort. It felt to us both that we were living through the worst few days of our lives. As she said afterwards, 'Within the space of twenty-four hours I discovered that I was pregnant with a new life growing inside me, and then I was told in the cruellest way that the father of my baby and the man I loved would soon be dead. It was the first time anyone had pointed out the full scale of what we were facing. It blew our minds.'

Neither of us wanted to stay there a moment longer, we couldn't wait to get away. All we wanted to do was go home, but as the news sank in on the journey we became even more anxious, and by the time we went to pick up Katy from school we were both so emotional we had to stop the car.

As the shock wore off and my anger began to set in I felt physically sick, as if I'd been kicked in the stomach. If I'd lost a limb or suffered shell shock, I'd have probably been nurtured to the end. Instead I felt like I was being abandoned.

The career I loved had just been terminated and I'd soon be unemployed – and possibly unemployable. The Army wasn't even going to support the bike ride I'd been dreaming about for years. On top of it all, Vicky continued to talk about keeping our baby, which could one day face the same terrible diagnosis.

Still shaken, I tried to reason with her and explain my point of view. 'It's not that I don't love you or wouldn't want to have a kid with you, Vicks. I just don't think it would be fair to bring a baby into this right now. I already have two children living with the threat of it hanging over them. I don't want to put another one through that too.'

She sobbed and sobbed but between her tears she said, 'I can take a test. We can get the foetus tested first.'

I sighed. 'I suppose, but then what?'

'Well, even if it tests positive, by the time he or she is forty, there'll be a cure.' It was a sentence she was to repeat frequently.

'Yeah, maybe.'

Wiping her eyes and placing a protective hand on her belly, she said something then that really broke my heart. Taking my hand, she said, 'I've just found out that I'm going to lose you, Chris, and I can't even bear to think about it. Five minutes of amazing versus nothing is one thing, but I never really thought that we'd have such a short time together.'

I began to tell her that I understood, but she wasn't finished.

'After you've gone, this baby will be the only part of you that I'll have left – something I can touch and hold and still love. Please don't take that away from me.'

Nodding, I pulled her into my arms and thought of the line in *The Shawshank Redemption*, my all-time favourite film. The character Andy Dufresne, played by Tim Robbins, speaks about hope as a good thing, adding, 'maybe the best of things. And no good thing ever dies.'

If in doubt – hope.

12

'Someday you will find the one who will watch every sunrise with you until the sunset of your life.'

UNKNOWN

Dementia Adventure Diary, 12 November 2015, Raleigh, North Carolina

The perfect song on my playlist for travelling through Florida and some of the Southern states with their five-star hotels, fancy houses and super yachts was Jessie J's 'Price Tag', with its line: *Why is everybody so obsessed? Money can't buy us happiness.* Never a truer word was spoken.

My video sitrep from the Florida Keys showed Shirley basking in the sunshine in front of crystal blue waters and a smattering of expensive vessels. 'There's thousands of yachts here,' I commented. 'It reeks of poverty – not!' In a happy mood I reported that I was still alive and well and looking forward to the end game of being in Toronto just before Christmas. I wrapped up with, 'If in doubt – buy a yacht. If you've got enough money anyway!'

My school chum Rachel commented: 'Bloody love you, you amazing man.' Vicky quipped that Shirley had become my Wilson, a reference to the film *Castaway* with Tom Hanks in which he becomes unreasonably attached to a Wilson basketball and starts to think of it as a person. She wasn't far from the truth. 'Keep pedalling, soldier,' she added. 'You've got a flight to catch!'

The thought of being on that plane home in only five weeks' time was quite staggering to me. Vicks had asked me to count how many rotations of my pedals I did in an average mile and then estimated that I must have done over six million pedal turns so far. I had also cycled almost 14,000 miles through sub-zero temperatures and blistering 120-plus degree heat. Even though that was me she was talking about, I couldn't quite get my head around it.

In spite of all its wealth, Florida was the land of punctures. Of the nine I experienced on my whole trip, seven were there, including the loss of an inner tube. The humidity also caused me some serious problems, affecting all my electrical leads and, crucially, preventing me from updating my position or charging up my devices. I bought some portable battery chargers, but they only had a limited life and I couldn't afford to keep buying more.

It didn't help that I accidentally left my tracker on continuously in a town called Lakeland, which meant that it sent far too many pings and used up all my credit. After that I had to go into 'ping rationing' and set it up to only transmit every twelve hours to save money. This meant that people couldn't follow me so easily on my Yellow-brick tracker map, but that couldn't be helped.

At one campsite somewhere in Florida I came across a German couple who had a far better system of charging their devices, something I really wish I'd known about before I set off. They had little dynamos attached to their bikes so that every turn of the pedal created electricity and gave them enough power to keep their devices full of juice. Clever Germans. If I ever did a major bike ride again, that was the one thing I'd do differ-ently. Oh, and be slightly better prepared for the wildlife. It was at that same campsite near a creek after a late night visit to do my ablutions that I wandered back to my tent by torchlight and thought I heard something. Panning my torch around, I spotted two red eyes staring back at me. They belonged to a large alligator three metres away. I very nearly had to rush straight back to the loo!

Carrying on up through Miami, I rode past Cape Canaveral with sadly no time to stop and visit the Kennedy Space Center, somewhere I have always wanted to go. As kids in Bollin Road Primary we were shown old footage of Neil Armstrong walking on the moon and it blew my mind. None of it felt real, and I think that was the first time in my life that I realised that we humans can achieve the impossible if we put our minds to it. Visiting the site from where man was first launched to the stars was high up my bucket list, but not now, not with Shirley in tow, and definitely not in a Lycra onesie.

Want to fly to the moon, Staff Graham?

Yes, sir! Tomorrow, sir! One question, though – how come we can get man to the moon but we haven't found a cure for dementia?

I was also close to Daytona Beach and would have loved to linger and watch some of its famed motorsports, but time was against me – in more ways than one. I pushed on near the border with Georgia, the 'Peach State', where I can faithfully report that the ripe peaches were delicious. Then I pressed on through busy Jacksonville, hotbed of the American Civil War, before crossing into South and then North Carolina, where I especially loved the *Gone with the Wind* mansions I whizzed past in places like Savannah and historic Charleston. Somewhere along a highway I came across an English pub with a red phone box and a double decker bus and that made me feel really homesick, especially when I found it was shut. I also spotted a medical facility named the John Graham Centre, so I stopped to take a photograph and pay a silent tribute to my late father. I remembered the Spanish moss with its own strange beauty that drips from the trees like an old man's beard from when I was in the Carolinas before. This time, though, the main thing dripping from the trees was rain.

The further north I pushed towards Raleigh, the cooler it became and the more layers I began to add. I feared how wintry it might be by the time I got to Washington and New York in December. Maybe I should have slowed down further back, as we'd always planned, so that I wouldn't be hitting those cities until the spring. Oh well, it was too late now.

I wasn't a stranger to cycling in inclement weather. The previous November, whilst I was still working through my resettlement period, I'd been asked by the PRU to take part in a week-long charity bike ride from Liverpool to commemorate the centenary of the First World War in aid of the charity Help for Heroes. Accompanied by a few of the lads from Headley Court, we stopped at war memorials along the way to lay wreaths, ending up in Yorkshire on Remembrance Sunday and the 100th anniversary of the outbreak of the First World War. There were a lot of hills and the weather was often brutal, but each day's ride was relatively short compared to my Dementia Adventure – due in part to the disabilities of some of my fellow cyclists. I'm so glad we did it and it felt even more important to pay homage to the fallen in my final year in the military.

I spent much of 2014 travelling with comrades, or still at the Army's beck and call, while I served out my notice. In March I'd flown to Bavaria on Exercise Snow Warrior, a ten-day ski course for disabled personnel run by ex-squaddies, as part of something called Battle Back Headley Court. As a proficient skier since before my days in Norway and with all my limbs intact, I was far better off than the less physically able and it was great to be doing something sporting and positive again. The conditions were ideal and the weather so good that five of us even stripped off for a cheeky bare-buttocks shot at the top of a mountain.

I also spent some time at the Royal British Legion facility at the Battle Back Centre, based at the Lilleshall National Sports Centre in the West Midlands. There I was delighted to bump into my first cousin John Stubbs, a competitive archer who won gold in the 2008 Paralympic Games. The son of my mum's elder sister May, John lost a leg and became wheelchair-bound after a car accident in his twenties, but he went on to represent Britain internationally in archery and be awarded an MBE. We don't do things by halves in our family.

I flew to Bulgaria to visit another mate who'd recently bought a house there and helped him with some building work. Then, in May, I joined another military group doing a battlefield tour of Belgium which included a visit to the Menin Gate Memorial to the Missing in Ypres. I was humbled by the nightly gathering of those wishing to honour the almost 55,000 men commemorated there and to hear a lone bugler play the Last Post – a tradition upheld since 1928. At 'Mud Corner', where German and British soldiers in no man's land had agreed a truce and downed weapons to sing carols and play a game of football on Christmas Eve, 1918, I took photos and found myself close to tears at the wholesale slaughter of so many young men.

Even though the Queen wouldn't have me in her service for much longer, I still had to obey orders and be a part of the family that I was being severed from before my time. The powers-that-be were also trying to prepare me for Civvy Street and advise me on what I should be organising regarding my personal affairs. At their suggestion, my sisters Lizzie and Angie, along with Neil Deadman, drove to see me in Headley Court to discuss drawing up power-of-attorney documents and working out what I wanted for my end-of-life care. I'm not very good at having those kinds of difficult conversations, though. A few forms were signed but nothing was settled.

Vicky and I were still trying to decide what was best for our unborn child. We talked it through endlessly, but I couldn't change how I felt and was still intent on trying to persuade her to terminate the pregnancy if the baby tested positive for the gene. I sensed her misgivings, though, and pro-mised to give her every opportunity to explore all possibilities before we made a final decision – together. Knowing that there would only be a short window in which to test the foetus *in utero* before we had to decide, she booked an appoint-ment with a midwife and asked her GP to refer her to a geneticist.

The doctors explained that she'd have two options for testing. The first, at around nine weeks, was called CVS (chorionic villi sampling), and would involve inserting a needle into the womb to draw off blood from the placenta and sending it off for DNA testing. The second was amniocentesis, which siphoned amniotic fluid and for which Vicky had to be at least fifteen weeks pregnant. There was a risk that merely having the tests could cause a miscarriage and by the time the results were analysed and returned to the hospital we'd only have a couple of weeks to go ahead with a termination – if that was what we decided. To her surprise, Vicks was informed that in a handful of cases termination can be performed right up to full term, and that a foetus with my PSEN1 gene fell into this category.

Vicky was horrified when they told her what the procedure involved. Even the earlier termination was no longer done under general anaesthetic. At eleven weeks, when the results would be known, that option was too late. Instead it would involve taking medication to induce contractions to expel the developing baby. If we decided to terminate at a later stage, it was even worse. The doctors would perform what is known as a surgical two-stage abortion, in which they'd inject the baby's heart with a needle to kill it and then induce labour to make Vicky give birth to our dead child.

She came home crying and told me she couldn't possibly go through with that. 'There's a fifty per cent chance our baby is completely healthy and doesn't even have the gene!' she said. 'What if we killed him or her and then doctors found a cure in a few years' time? How could we live with ourselves and the image of our stillborn baby in our minds reminding us forever what we'd done?'

Once I heard that, I knew she was right. It was a no-brainer. There was no way either of us could do that to our innocent child and, without specifically voicing it to each other, we both knew then that we would go ahead and have our baby. When, though, we asked the doctors if we could have the genetics test anyway – and soon if possible so that at least we knew either way – we came up against a whole new set of problems and our battle with the hospital ethics board began. The powers-that-be argued that if the test was positive, then – ethically – we should agree to destroy our baby. They claimed that otherwise, long before they were legally entitled to know themselves, our son or daughter would grow up with their parents knowing they had the gene, and that could potentially affect their childhood.

Vicks was as furious as I was, and she told them, 'You're talking as if our baby has already got the gene when the chances are it's perfectly healthy. That's all we want to know. And besides, in forty years' time there'll undoubtedly be a cure!' Despite our protestations, they refused to give us the test if we refused to sign the documents agreeing to an abortion. Just as with the decision to discharge me from the Army on medical grounds, there was no right of appeal.

Emotionally drained by the catalogue of disasters that seemed to be befalling us in quick succession, Vicky and I decided to take a break and drive to Stonehenge for Summer Solstice on 21 June. We're not hippies or Druids, but sunrises have always held a special allure to me, and I was delighted that Vicks felt the same way about them and wanted to feature them as part of a special photography project. We hoped that a few days away together on our own after we'd been bombarded with so much bad news would help clear our heads.

Just as we were preparing to set off on 20 June, the telephone rang. It was my stepfather Eric, calling to tell us that Mum had suffered a stroke at home and was in hospital. It was minor and she'd rallied at first, he said, but then she had a second stroke which rendered her unconscious, and the doctors said there was nothing more they could do.

The memory of standing by her bed at Wythenshawe Hospital will remain with me for ever. Dorothy Graham was sixty-six and hadn't had an easy time on this earth. Born into poverty and struggling for much of her life, she'd lost Dad far too young and in horrible circumstances, and then tried to cope as best she could in the midst of her grief. Some may have criticised her for sending her boys away, but the way I looked at it was that if I hadn't gone to the children's home, I might never have joined the Army.

When I arrived at the hospital with Vicky, I quickly introduced her to the rest of my family. It didn't seem possible that they'd not even had a chance to meet yet, but then so much had happened in the previous few months. The last time I'd seen my sisters was in early March when I'd been staying in Manchester with Lizzie. My children Natalie and Marcus flew in for a long weekend and we had a big family get-together in a local hotel. Vicky hadn't accompanied me as we'd only just met and it was all too new. Mum had been so happy that day, relishing the rarity of having four of her five children around her. Tony wasn't well enough to come, sadly, but most of the grandchildren were there and it was a very happy – if noisy – night. We had some group photos taken and then we kissed goodbye.

Now it was time for the final farewell and none of us felt ready. Sixty-six was no age at all and I think we'd expected that tireless worker, mother and grandmother to go on for ever. Vicks and I sat around her bedside with Lizzie and Angie, our half-sister Alison and Eric, listening to her breathing become more laboured as each of us struggled with our emotions.

Hours later, when everyone else had gone home and an exhausted Eric was fast asleep in the corner, I sat with Vicks at the end of the bed and thought back to all the trouble I'd given Mum as a nipper. I rarely did as I was told and spent most of my childhood running wild in the woods or down by the river. Even when I was home, I managed to scald myself or get wedged in the bedhead. Poor woman, she'd had such a time of it and all the hard knocks had made her brittle and often uncompromising. In her latter years, though, she'd grown softer and wiser and I was so grateful that she and I had made our peace. There was nothing to regret and nothing left unsaid.

Except perhaps one thing.

Squeezing her hand, I leaned forward and whispered, 'You're going to be a grandmother again, Mum. My girlfriend Vicky and I are having a baby.' Saying those words out loud galvanised the news in my mind. I not only knew we were definitely going to keep the baby, but I wanted it more

221

than anything else in the world.

Mum's breathing changed and she gave a little sigh and I was convinced then that she would wake up to congratulate us, but she never did. Exhausted by the day's events, we eventually drove to a nearby hotel to grab a few hours' sleep. Almost as soon as we reached our room at around 2 a.m., though, Eric rang to tell us that Mum had just passed away.

Back at the hospital, it was hard to believe Mum was dead and not just sleeping, she looked so peaceful. We were all devastated. Trying to buoy up my sisters, I said quietly, 'Vicks is pregnant,' and watched their tear-stained faces light up. They were thrilled, hugging us both. And they were wholeheartedly behind our decision to go ahead with the pregnancy.

'There'll be a cure any day, Chris,' Lizzie told me, echoing Vicky's oft-repeated statement and delighted at the prospect of being an auntie again. Our unborn baby was the only beacon of light in that gloomy hospital room.

By the time we drove home from the hospital hours later, the sun was floating up over the horizon like a vast orange lantern burning the whole sky red. It was one of the most beautiful sunrises I had ever seen and, with tears in my eyes, I stopped the car and asked Vicks to take a photograph.

One week after my twenty-second anniversary of first joining the army in Chepstow in 1992, we gave Mum a simple send-off at Altrincham crematorium; the same place my father had been cremated thirty-three years earlier. Tony was with us, but I don't think he knew where he was or even appreciated the fact that Mum had died. I volunteered to be a pallbearer, having done it a few times for fellow soldiers over the years. Speaking from experience, I warned the others, 'Be careful. The coffin will be heavy. Don't drop her.'

To my shock and surprise, it was exactly the opposite. The coffin was so light there can't have been anything of her. There appeared to be no weight at all to show for all the burdens she had suffered in life.

Standing stiffly in the front row for the short service, I watched her disappear behind the curtain and couldn't quite believe that she was gone for ever. 'Bye Mum,' I whispered. 'Rest in peace.'

My sisters and I had agreed to try to celebrate her life rather than mourn her death and part of me was grateful that she hadn't lived long enough to see Tony worsen and die, or watch me slowly decline. She'd been through too much with Dad to have to witness us both succumbing to the same fate.

Together as a family we said our farewells and celebrated her life in epic style. Not long after her funeral I presented each of my siblings with a gift. It was a printed canvas of the special sunrise Vicky had photographed for me the morning Mum died; a permanent memento of a remarkable woman.

If in doubt – watch the sun come up.

13

'Friends show their love
in times of trouble, not in happiness.'

EURIPIDES

Dementia Adventure Diary, 15 November 2015, Washington, DC

As I pushed on north towards the finishing line, I was very relieved to be on the final leg but utterly miserable much of the time too. The cold, wet, windy weather was reminiscent of my first leg in Ontario. I was missing Vicks terribly. And, with less than a hundred quid in my bank account, I was ready to go home.

The one song that Vicky and I think of as 'ours' is 'Iris' by the Goo Goo Dolls, and it was a frequent chart-topper on my playlist, especially as I cycled the east coast of America. With its talk of being unable to fight the inevitable it feels somehow tailor-made for us, especially the prophetic line, *When everything's made to be broken, I just want you to know who I am.* Now if that doesn't tug on the heartstrings, then I don't know what does.

There were a few major milestones to get through before I was reunited with Vicks, though, and my biggest two were Washington, DC and Manhattan. Riding through cities had become my greatest dread on this trip. The lanes were narrow, there was a terrifying amount of traffic and – at twelve feet end to end with the trailer – Shirley was a nightmare to manoeuvre on roads jam-packed with intimidating trucks, buses, cars and pedestrians. In between keeping my eyes peeled for street signs, I had to pedal across busy intersections, make hazardous right turns, negotiate contraflows and watch out for signals. Being in an urban jungle made it far too risky for me to refer to the satnav all the time, so Vicky had to talk me through the busiest areas in my ear, and the rest of the time I had to rely on my wits – a dangerous precedent in my case.

Somehow, and by the skin of my teeth, I made it to Arlington, Virginia, on the outskirts of Washington and managed to find the motel where I was meeting up with Pete Davies. It was so great to see his smiling face. From the moment I'd told him I had dementia in 2013 and then outlined my plans for the ride, he'd expressed his full support. 'I won't be able to do the whole thing around America with you, but I can join you for part of it,' he said. 'We've got shipmates we can stay with in Washington or Calgary so let's aim for either of those.'

Several other friends had offered to come with me but I knew that, for most, it wasn't feasible. Who amongst them could realistically afford to take extended time off work and pay for themselves and their bikes to be flown across the Atlantic from England just to ride alongside me for a few days? My mate Neil had been in just that situation. He had always intended to come with me from the get-go, but that was in the summer of

2014 when he was single and not yet in the job he'd since found for himself. My time in Headley Court going through the military medical mill had delayed everything, so that by the time I was set to leave in April 2015, he was working full-time and had a girlfriend who was pregnant. It would have been a massive ask for him to drop everything and join me and – although gutted at first – I completely understood when he told me he couldn't.

Pete was in a different position and coming to the end of his Army career. Man of his word that he was, he agreed to ride the one hundred and thirty or so miles between Washington, DC and Philadelphia with me, before taking a train back to DC and flying home. He even bought his own bike and panniers especially for the trip, although I'm not sure he would say that the effort and the expense were worth it in the end. It peed down and was freezing the whole time he was with me, even when we chilled for a while to give him time to 'get over his jet lag'. What I didn't know until later was that Vicky had made Pete promise to persuade me to stay put for a couple of days to give me some enforced rest, because she was worried I was pushing myself too hard.

Although I was keen to get on, I really enjoyed our time in the US capital. I also managed to tick a few things off on my bucket list, with visits to the White House, the Lincoln Memorial, the Tomb of the Unknowns, the famous Iwo Jima Memorial (officially the US Marine Corps War Memorial), and Arlington Cemetery, where we paid our respects to those US servicemen who died in the Second World War. We stayed at the home of our former shipmate Kev Pellington, who hosted us fantastically. He worked at the British Embassy, where we were taken to meet the Defence Attaché, Major General Richard Cripwell, who gave us a very warm welcome and publicly referred to my journey as 'inspirational'. Later that night Pete posted a photo of me and Kev in the bar with the tongue-in-cheek caption, 'In training.'

On 16 November, in matching red and black Lycra, Pete and I set off together on our bikes headed for Baltimore, forty miles north-west, where I was due to rendezvous with a BBC crew and veteran television presenter Angela Rippon to film a documentary about living with dementia to be broadcast on my return.

Pete was as fit as a flea and had done a bit of training for the trip, but he wasn't a cyclist and had only really started riding a bike the week before he flew out to join me. I, meanwhile, was fully conditioned and always going to be faster than him, even pulling a trailer. I was also impatient to crack on to the next stop, so I'm sure he thought I was a bit of a nutter as I flew off ahead of him with hardly a glance behind me. I didn't expect him to keep up with me but he did his best, even in such inclement conditions.

The BBC had booked us a room each at the Ramada Inn, Ellicott City on the outskirts of Baltimore (the room was far swankier than anything I'd stayed in up until that point) and when we arrived – two men in matching Lycra – the receptionist made an assumption and gave us a double room. We had to laugh when we saw the queen-size divan and we called up Vicky lying side by side on the luxurious deep-filled bedding. 'Well, Pete is ready, willing and able...' I reasoned, jokingly.

Poor Pete, Vicky should have warned him what it was like sleeping with me. I always drop off within minutes but then I have hallucinations and all sorts of crazy moments where I don't know where I am or who I'm with. It often takes me several minutes to get back into the zone. One night with her, I lifted my head off the pillow and started twisting it violently from left to right. 'What are you doing?' Vicks asked, sitting bolt upright and turning on the light.

'Training for the pentathlon,' I replied, as if it was the most normal thing in the world. Another time, I jumped up to run my hands all along the wall, the wardrobe and the curtains. 'Go back to sleep,' I told her. 'I'm just checking the perimeter.' Needless to say, she couldn't doze off again for ages.

When Pete got up to use the loo in our Baltimore hotel room and came back into the room bleary-eyed, I leapt out of bed and screamed: 'Who the bloody hell are you?'

'It's me. Pete – you plonker!' he replied. I don't remember a thing about it but he said it took him a minute or two to calm me down until my addled brain was able to register the information that for the first time in months there was someone else sharing my billet.

Filming started early the next morning and – both of us being strangers to the vagaries of a documentarian's schedule – we were surprised at how long the crew took to record what would probably translate to only a few minutes' worth of airtime. Pete sat around for hours inside in a warm café chatting to the crew with tea and cake on tap (it's a tough old life), while I was filmed cycling up and down steep hills for what felt like a hundred takes. It seemed to last for ever, especially when we were both itching to get on with the trip. It was well worth it in the end, though – it was a new and good experience and they treated us very well.

Released back into the wild and the 'Free State' of Maryland, we set off towards Philadelphia, Pennsylvania, in driving rain. Cold and drenched through, we managed thirty-seven miles before stopping for a burger, and then another thirty or so before we stopped at a motel to dry out for the night. After a hotdog, Pete posted a video in which he claimed, 'To say it's raining is an understatement. I don't think I've ever seen rain like it.' Our friend and former fitness instructor, Swifty, commented drily: 'If it's not raining, you ain't training!'

Setting off early the next morning and relying on my navigational expertise as I rode several yards ahead of him, Pete blindly followed me to Philadelphia airport, which was never the plan – although I refused to admit I was lost. If in doubt – deny everything. Then, after we found our way back to where we were meant to be, I accidentally led him through a ghetto and the docks before taking him up onto the seven-lane Benjamin Franklin suspension bridge spanning the mighty Delaware River. It was hammering down with rain and blowing a gale, which meant that it wasn't the greatest view in the world, and I heard Pete grumble, 'Well, this is quality.' His face reminded me of Karl Pilkington from *An Idiot Abroad*.

He said later, 'I don't like heights and, although I'd trust Chris with my life, he scared the pants off me that day. He was like a Ninja. Imagine cycling the Firth of Forth Bridge in the worst weather shortly after riding through a ghetto – two white lads with expensive bikes. I'd gone to enjoy the great outdoors and all I saw was rain and docks.'

Even I have to admit that bridge was dangerous. We were both clipped into our bikes and liable to be blown or knocked off any minute. I think that was the first time Pete realised just how high up we were and that cyclists weren't allowed. He was crapping himself. 'You've illegally taken me onto this bridge!' he cried. 'You're trying to kill me!' We took some crazy photographs up there.

He admitted later, 'I was scared from the moment we started to the minute I finished.' He was also a bit concerned by how often I repeated myself when discussing things and how confused I sometimes seemed, asking him to remind me what day it was or where we were. He witnessed my OCD routines morning and night, when I would check and recheck my kit two or three times over to make sure I hadn't forgotten anything. 'It only made me appreciate even more what an incredible thing Chris was doing and how lonely it was out there on his own,' he said afterwards.

We stopped for the night at a motel with a view of the bridge we'd almost died on and woke up to better, brighter weather, which lifted our spirits enormously. Sadly, reaching Philly – home of the

American Declaration of Independence and the Liberty Bell – sounded the death knell for my time with Pete, who had to get back to being a warrant officer (first class) in the British Army for the final month of his twenty-four years' service in the regiment.

He was due to be 'dined out' in style back at South Cerney, with a chance to wear full mess kit and hear his commanding officer say great things about him in front of all his mates at a big send-off party. It was something I'd always expected to happen to me too when it was time to hang up my boots, but since Aldershot I wanted none of it. I was very happy for Pete, though, and his generosity to me had been unbelievable. Not only had he shelled out hundreds of pounds to come and support me on the road, but once he arrived – and knowing how short of money I was – he refused to let me pay for a thing.

On a bright and frosty morning outside our motel the day he was due to head back south, I posted a video of the two of us and publicly thanked him for his support. When he pretended to be crying, I commented: 'Dry your eyes, Princess.' An hour later, at a major crossroads in the city, Pete turned left towards the Amtrak train station and I turned right towards New York. Waving him goodbye, I felt genuine emotion at seeing him go. It had been such a blast having him there in support, and as I said at the time – and as I've repeated endlessly since – 'Pete Davies is an awesome, awesome man.'

Bless him, he posted that he'd never forget coming on my Dementia Adventure with me, adding, 'The best thing of all was being there as promised for a great friend – LEGEND Chris.' Back in England he wrote, 'Recently I was privileged to share a small part of the 16,000-mile epic challenge that my friend Chris Graham is undertaking in the name of charity; such a selfless sacrifice by such a great human being. Please show your support by either following his progress or sponsoring one of the two charities. If you live on any part of the route Boston–Toronto please offer him a smiling face, a cup of tea, or a simple act of kindness. Many thanks for making me believe in humanity again.'

Thanks, Boss.

On 25 November, a few days after he left me, and a month to the day before Christmas, I received a much-needed boost with the fantastic news that I had won the Sporting Charity Challenge of the Year in the Pride of Sport Awards 2015. Vicks got to spend the night all dressed up in Grosvenor House Hotel for that one, and this time she wasn't late. 'Well done babe,' she wrote online. 'So bloody proud I could burst!' Her picture of my glass trophy sparked dozens of comments and good wishes from friends and strangers alike.

Sometimes when I hear what people say about me, or how they congratulate me on what I've achieved with this ride, I find it difficult to accept their praise. This challenge was something I always wanted to do – for me as much as anyone else – and I felt and believed that it was a great privilege to do so. I was in a unique and enviable position to be able to take a year out and use my

Army pay-off to fund it and, with time running out for me, I was grateful that I was still well enough to make the attempt.

Ever since 2010, I had been given regular and frequent reminders of what I was facing and how medicine would eventually shape my future. Having been identified because of Tony's health issues as the unlucky recipient of this faulty gene, my sisters and I were invited to take part in the global familial Alzheimer's disease trial with the handful of families around the world who were facing the same challenges. When you add up my three kids, Tony's two boys, and four others in our wider family, there are nine children currently facing the possibility of inheriting the 'daft gene', so the hope was that, once on board, we might be offered trial drugs before anyone else.

It is a sad fact of life that the majority of patients with late-onset 'sporadic' Alzheimer's only come to the attention of specialists once major symptoms have developed, at which point the disease has taken hold and is much harder to treat. By assessing people like me before that point of no return, scientists and doctors can chart the earliest signs of the disease. In theory, they can then track its progress right up to my death, and within a relatively short period of time compared to a 'normal' Alzheimer's patient. This may also allow them to monitor the impact of new therapies at close quarters and use that information to decode other dementias. In time, they hope to diagnose the disease much earlier and come up with something that could make a difference, ideally before symptoms have even started.

What I didn't appreciate at first was that my agreement to take part would involve becoming a human guinea pig. I was placed under the overall supervision of Professor Nick Fox and his team, including Dr Philip Weston, at the Dementia Research Centre, University College Hospital (UCH), London, where in 1991 – ten years after my father died – the first FAD gene was identified after painstaking and laborious investigation of individual chromosomes. Alzheimer's was first identified by German doctor Alois Alzheimer in 1906, and by the 1930s doctors recognised that in certain families the disease appeared to be inherited, and that family members could get it as early as thirty if they were unlucky enough to have the faulty dominant gene.

Professor Fox and his colleagues now work together as part of an international research partnership known as the Dominantly Inherited Alzheimer Network (DIAN), based at Washington University School of Medicine in St Louis, Missouri. He told us that the disease seems to present itself in a very consistent way. 'If in a family with a particular mutation people got it in their fifties then you are most at risk in your fifties, in a pattern that repeats itself and breeds true. People have exactly the same gene, which produces exactly the same defect, which produces exactly the same protein abnormality, which will produce the same changes in the brain. But even in families where things are very similar, you might get someone with an onset at thirty-five and a sibling with an onset at forty-five, so there is some variation.'

Under his supervision at UCH, and at Addenbrooke's in Cambridge, I was regularly poked and prodded, tested and grilled. Lizzie and Angie were as well to begin with, but they had to drop out because of the time it all took and their family commitments. Unlike Army interrogation techniques, I was encouraged to give much more than my name, rank and serial number. The most unpleasant parts of the trial were having lumbar punctures to draw off cerebral spinal fluid to check for proteins and cell destruction. They'd inject dye into my veins while I was in a claustrophobic brain scanner so that they could examine the extent of the amyloid proteins in my brain. I also had umpteen blood tests and CAT scans in noisy machines with terrible music playing. Haven't these people heard of Ed Sheeran?

Professor Fox says the work he does with familial versions of the disease humbles and moves him every day. He sympathises with those families who actively try to cover up their medical history to protect the next generation, blaming everything from the menopause to shell shock, as my relatives may have done. 'It is such a burden for children to know that there is something inherited. People also worry about the chances of finding a partner and can suffer from depression as they approach the age when a parent or sibling began to develop symptoms.'

His team has been responsible for some groundbreaking results from their twenty-plus years of research, chiefly that changes in the brain structure of someone with Alzheimer's can appear up to five years before any symptoms develop. 'Our brains shrink gradually as we age but what we found was particular shrinkage specifically in memory areas early on. This started before symptoms and then year-on-year accelerated and spread to other parts of the brain, giving people up to five times the normal loss for their age.'

This meant that the general assumption that the FAD gene was 'switched on' and that patients suddenly 'fell off a cliff' was incorrect. 'The amazing thing is that this opens a window for intervention,' he added. 'The ideal time would be when you have some evidence of disease but you haven't had any destruction because of it. If we can treat people when they are pre-symptomatic then that is the best option, because most people would rather be treated when they are well than when they are bedbound and mute.'

He said this is especially true in early-onset dementia because the body whose brain is being ravaged by this 'ruthless disease' is often young, fit and healthy, and can survive in that state for longer than someone elderly. 'These very rare families have contributed hugely, disproportionately, to the research. Most of our treatment of dementia will have come from our knowledge of what these genes have told us about what they do.'

The first waves of therapies using antibodies to attack the proteins began while I was on my bike ride, so I missed my chance to trial that one, but I may be added to the next wave. I was certainly more than happy to do the tests and try the drugs if it meant shedding some light on the disease and helping the next generation – including ours.

The most boring part of it for me involved what

I called the mind games, where I'd sit in a room with a specialist for virtually a whole day doing puzzles and playing with shapes using something akin to children's wooden building blocks. Then there were the mental agility tests, where they might show me eighty or so photographs of people with different expressions on their faces and ask me, 'How do you think this person is feeling, Chris?'

'Happy,' I'd reply. 'Angry,' or 'Sad.'

When we'd worked our way through the entire set of photos they'd show me several of them again and ask me if I'd seen that face before. There'd be steam coming out of my ears by the time I'd finished and I'd be more than ready for a breath of fresh air and a brew.

Even though Vicky was pregnant and physically uncomfortable, she came along with me to one of my assessments in London so that she could get an understanding of what these pioneering scientists were trying to achieve. She soon realised how boring it was and how – every now and again – I had a mischievous urge to liven things up a little.

Sitting to one side in the office where I was being tested, Vicky watched as I sat opposite my latest inquisitor with his questions on a clipboard, which he foolishly laid flat on the table in front of him. Within seconds of him beginning the test, she realised that I was secretly reading the answers upside down from his list. Winking at her as she stifled a giggle, I carried on giving answers Einstein would have been proud of while he scribbled down my answers on a separate piece of paper.

Once the test was over, he looked up with a smile and said, 'Well done, Chris! You did a lot better this time.'

Vicks snorted laughter so loudly out of her nose that we both looked up in surprise. 'Sorry,' she said, shrugging innocently and hardly daring to catch my eye. 'It's my hormones. I think I need to be excused to use the bathroom for a moment.' I could hear her laughing all the way down the corridor.

This Johnny Gurkha wasn't really cheating, sir. I was simply doing what I'd been trained to do and using my initiative.

If in doubt – adapt and overcome.

14

'Since the day of my birth, my death
began its walk.
It is walking toward me, without hurrying.'
JEAN COCTEAU

Dementia Adventure Diary, 26 November 2015, Boston, Massachusetts

Most people are never forced to consider the manner or timing of their death. It's a very human reaction to choose not to think about it, or even to deny the inevitable for fear it might tempt fate. That's probably why so many people die without having written a will.

My closest brush with death was in 1995 in Bosnia, when the truck in which I was a passenger lost control on a slippery hill in the winter and almost fell into a sixty-metre ravine not far from Split. 'Fuck! We're dead!' I yelled, gripping my seat, but the driver, Dom, somehow managed to stop us sliding into the abyss and steered the lorry, with its heavy container on the back, into a sheer rock face instead.

Trucks seem to have it in for me. Cycling through Jersey City and the so-called 'Garden State' on my way to New York, I was nearly killed four times by metal monsters that came uncomfortably close. Struggling not to be sucked into their slipstream, I truly thought I might end up under the wheels. Feeling more than a bit panicky, I stopped to catch my breath and post a video online in which I sounded far more jovial than I felt: 'I don't know if I will survive this city but, if I don't, I'll leave all my vast debt to anyone I know.'

The risks only worsened by the time I reached Manhattan, and I fully expected to die in the shadow of the Empire State Building. New York was one of the places I'd been determined to include on my trip as it is the home of one of the research teams investigating FAD and I hoped to drop in and say hello. But plans are what you make when someone's laughing, because not only did I never get to stay anywhere near the centre, but I was on such a tight deadline that I had no time to stop.

Vicky had plotted my route through the city and come up with a brilliant plan to navigate me via the quieter, safer cycle routes rather than risk me being squashed on the busy streets. The trouble was, many of those paths ran through the city's parks and in the winter, most were closed at 7.30 p.m.

Forced back onto the main roads in the dark, I was tired, cold and hungry. I hadn't eaten for hours and I needed to get some food inside me and get my head down for the night. Somewhat grumpily, I found myself not far from the Hudson River and in a residential area, which was fine until I came to a junction where Vicky – thinking I was facing in the opposite direction – told me to take a left but inadvertently sent me right.

Obeying orders and in my tired, confused state, I found myself on the edge of a six-lane highway of fast-moving traffic. Being there was more terrifying than anything I'd ever experienced in my life.

'Bloody hell!' I cried above the noise of the vehicles that rocked Shirley and me each time they thundered past. There was virtually no hard shoulder and the cars and trucks were less than a foot away and flying past me at 60 mph. Sensing immediately that I could die and realising that it had to be illegal for me to be there, I dismounted and jumped over the barrier flanking the narrow hard shoulder, leaving poor Shirley stranded on the traffic side.

'Now what, Vicks?' I asked her on the phone, my nerves frayed. 'This is really bad. I don't think I'm going to get out of here alive.'

'Hang on, babes. I just need to figure out where you are,' she replied, desperately trying to reassure me. It was about 4 a.m. for her and I'm sure she was just as fatigued as I was. 'I think if you can get onto the next slip road, then five hundred metres the other side you'll be in the right neighbourhood.' I could tell she was trying to stay calm and keep me focused.

I didn't know where she meant. 'There's no way I can cross to the other side!' I cried, exasperated. It felt as if I stood there for an hour breathing hard and waiting for inspiration, or for her to come up with a better plan. I have no idea how long it really was, but after what seemed an age I saw a New York cop car slow down as it drove past on the other side of the highway, with the armed officer in the driver's seat staring at me ferociously.

'Oh God, the busies are here, Vicks! I think they're going to come back around and arrest me!'

Looking frantically around me in the dark, my eyes followed the steep tree-lined embankment behind me to what I then realised was almost certainly the slip road she'd intended me to be on. 'Come on, soldier,' I chastised myself, and started to pull my panniers one by one. 'Forward march!'

It took me four trips, scrabbling up the rough bank and scratching my hands and knees in the process, to get them to the top. Then I slid back down again and unhitched my trailer. I lifted it up over the barrier before doing the same for Shirley. By the time the police came back around, just as I'd suspected they would, I was hiding in the bushes. Even though they used their flashlights to scan the embankment as they crawled past, they couldn't see hide nor hair of me. Which is just as well. I don't think I'd have much enjoyed a night in a New York police cell.

Vicky was with me all the way as I tried to get my rig to where it needed to be. She heard me puffing and panting as I hauled everything to the top of the hill, and then she heard me suddenly say, 'Oh hello. All right mate?'

'Who's that?' she asked, worried.

I couldn't answer her immediately because the two potheads I'd discovered smoking cannabis by the side of the road would have heard me. Hoping that they were as harmless as they looked, I said, 'Can you give me a hand with my kit, please?'

To my surprise, they rose to their feet (a bit unsteadily) and did exactly as I asked, lifting my panniers, trailer and bike over the second barrier at the top of the hill. I reassembled my rig and cycled away from them as fast as my weary legs would carry me.

Back on track, Vicks told me, 'Okay, panic over. Now let me get you to a motel.'

I followed her directions but soon began to notice that I wasn't in the best part of town. 'It seems a bit dodgy round here, babes,' I muttered. 'In fact, it looks like the sort of place I could be mugged.' Staring down at my device I realised that she'd directed me to the heart of the Bronx.

'All right, don't worry,' she replied, with telltale tension in her voice. 'There's a motel two miles up the road. I'll direct you to it.'

I eventually got there at about 11 p.m. and hurried in, anxious about leaving Shirley outside on her own. 'Excuse me,' I asked the receptionist, who was furiously chewing gum. 'Have you got a room?'

'Only until one a.m.,' she replied, without even looking up.

'One a.m.? But I need to get my head down!'

Listening in, Vicky realised with horror that she'd directed me to a house of ill repute, so she said quickly, 'It's okay, Chris. Get out of there. There's another place across the street. It's called the Friendly something.'

I did as I was told and lugged Shirley up the steps, with what felt like the last of my strength, before wearily asking the same question.

'Maximum three hours,' came the deadpan reply. When I looked round I spotted a chalkboard with the 'menu' of Friendly specials on offer that night.

'Bloody hell, Vicks!' I cried. 'What have you brought me to now?

'Forget that place,' she instructed. 'There's a couple more options...' As the next option had a flashing sign on the door offering Fantasy Rooms, I didn't even bother to ask, although by that point I was seriously considering taking anything. It might only be five minutes of amazing but at least I'd fall asleep with a smile. Needless to say, when Vicky eventually found me somewhere clean and safe to sleep that night where I wasn't going to be mugged, expected to have sex with a hooker, or be turfed out after two hours, I went out like a light.

Aside from the risk of being murdered in the Bronx or dying in a traffic accident, I have had to look death in the face far sooner than most, and that isn't something I'd wish on my worst enemy. Because of the defective gene that lurks inside my DNA, I've also been forced to consider something most people never have to think about – the possibility of taking the matter into my own hands.

This is especially true now that I have a much clearer understanding of how my father, aunt and cousin ended their days and am a reluctant witness to Tony's unhappy decline. In spite of my enduring hope that the doctors might miraculously discover a cure before I go completely daft, I'm in the unenviable position of knowing exactly what my fate will be – a slow death in a prison cell without doors. I would do almost anything to prevent that from happening, but even my bravado might fail me one day.

When Vicks suggested we sit down together and watch a BBC documentary called *How to Die*, about a Brit called Simon Binner who had motor neurone disease, I wasn't keen. Given the choice, like most people I'd rather not have to confront the stark truth. But this was a groundbreaking film about an extremely courageous man and his family, and we were both glad we watched it through until the end.

Simon was a successful businessman in his fifties when he was diagnosed with the condition, which went on to rob him of his speech and motor function. Relatively early on, he was adamant that he wanted to go to Switzerland for an assisted suicide. Although motor neurone disease is an awful thing to have, it does at least give sufferers the option to make that decision because they remain of sound mind to the end – unlike those of us with dementia, who lose all clarity. Even so, Simon's wife Debbie was very torn about his choice almost to the last day, but when he finally administered himself a lethal dose of anaesthetic, she, his friends and family were with him, holding his hand.

I rarely cry. But, seeing that, I lost it completely, and so did Vicks. We were both inconsolable at the thought of maybe having to go through the same thing one day ourselves, if I was even allowed the dignity of doing so. I almost can't imagine the enormous courage it would take to make the decision and then stick by it, even to the point of hosting a party and dinner to say goodbye to everyone you love. Or having the balls to take the dose that you know will terminate your life on this earth in a matter of minutes. Each time I visit Tony and see what kind of existence he has, however, that choice becomes far less difficult to understand.

If ever I were to consider assisted suicide, like Simon Binner I'd be faced with the terrible dilemma of when to do it. He set a date in his diary and tried to stick to it, but when that day came around, he was persuaded to postpone because his loved ones weren't ready and he still had some quality of life. The agonies he and his family went through as they debated exactly when he should kill himself were painful to witness. And then there's the whole question of having to fly to Switzerland to carry out the deed six hundred miles from home, because the law forbids assisted suicide in the UK.

If I were still a soldier I could have put a bullet in my head when the time came, but I'd still have to decide when that time was. After watching that remarkable documentary, I can see that there would always be a reason to postpone – Vicky's birthday perhaps, or mine; a milestone for the children, or the promise of a new drug I might be asked to trial. When is a good time to die? Is there one? And what about all those I'd leave behind – not just Vicky and my kids, but my sisters and all the rest of my family and friends. How would they feel if I killed myself?

'How to Die was an important film to watch,' Vicky said afterwards. 'It made us talk about the possibilities even if we choose never to consider them. All we want is for Chris to have as much normality and preserve his dignity for as long as possible. He deserves that. Nobody wants to think about dying or imagine how it might be when all dignity is lost, but sometimes it's good to have had that discussion at least.'

As far as I was concerned, the discussion was over – for now anyway. I'd file the memory of Simon and his incredible family away somewhere and, with any luck, I might even forget it. Up until the point where I felt that I was on the brink of losing all mental capacity, there was nothing I could do but keep focused on the positive and think about the future in very small packages.

Besides, I had so many positives to be thankful for, not least baby Dexter.

Vicky and I had settled on that name because we liked the sound of it and 'Dex' (it had nothing to do with the TV show about a serial killer, I promise). The name Oliver was the five-to-one favourite for a while – until I realised that he'd probably be called 'Ollie the Wally' at school. So we switched. It was always our intention to honour Tony too if we had a son, so his second name was Anthony. We hadn't picked a first name for a girl by the time we found out our baby would be a boy, but we had decided on the middle name Dorothy. Mum would have liked that.

Once we'd worked out Dexter's due date, 11 February 2015, Vicks and I planned everything so that I'd be home for his birth and spend the next two months helping out before I set off on my bike ride. There was much to organise in the months leading up to the big day and Vicks was working and studying for her diploma in photography at the same time. The subject of her first major course exhibition was 'Ruins', which was appropriate considering she was living with one! In true Vicky style, she not only gained her diploma, but was awarded a distinction.

She'd had a tricky first pregnancy with pre-eclampsia and something called polyhydramnios, which means that she produces too much amniotic fluid around the foetus. 'When your waters burst I'll get my surfboard out and we can ride the wave to the hospital!' I joked. Because of this excess fluid, she gained seven stone with Katy and then the baby came out sideways, which caused all sorts of problems including a life-threatening haemorrhage. With Dexter she gained five stone and that was still quite something to see. She'd be the first to admit she looked like a Spacehopper.

Her belly was so enormous that when she was

designing my website I had to kneel in front of her holding the laptop as she had no knees left to rest it on! Then the scans showed that our little Graham monkey was going to make it even more difficult for her by being a transverse breach, so a Caesarian section was decided upon as soon as she experienced the first twinges of labour. I'd been there at the births of both Natalie and Marcus – in Voss, Norway, and Cheltenham, Gloucestershire, respectively – and I fully intended to be there to personally welcome young Dexter into this world.

On 22 January, Vicky felt an almighty pain and we drove straight to the hospital. 'He's going to come tonight!' she told anyone who'd listen, but no one believed her and the doctors kept repeating that she wasn't dilated and had another few weeks to go. I went home to give Katy her tea, but Vicks had another contraction soon afterwards and rang to tell me, 'Get back here, Chris. Quick!'

I took one look at her lying on the hospital bed and announced, 'Yup. She's gonna blow!' But by 11 p.m. nothing had happened, so the medical team sent me home. Frustrated and in pain, Vicky ate a shepherd's pie at midnight. When the nurse came to collect her tray, she had another mighty contraction and then burst into tears. Within minutes she was in full-blown labour, yelling, 'Call Chris! Get him here now!'

My ability to sleep anywhere and extremely deeply is well chronicled. Even a grizzly bear rattling bins couldn't wake me in Ontario, remember. So when the telephone rang at 2 a.m. and a nurse woke me from my slumber to tell me Vicky had gone into labour, I thought it was a dream and slipped straight back to sleep. Vicks, meanwhile, was sucking on gas and air in order to get herself high enough to ignore the pain and refused to let the midwives do anything until I was by her side. She's stubborn that way.

'Call him again!' she screamed. 'He's fucking fallen back to sleep!'

A second phone call did the trick. I jumped into action and was in the car driving the thirty minutes to Oxford like Lewis Hamilton on steroids. I even overtook a police car but, thankfully, the officer didn't seem to notice. By the time I got to the hospital, Vicks was all prepped for the op in the delivery room and a nurse was standing with a gown held up for me to walk my arms straight into. With an elasticated cap on my head, I looked just like Del Boy – a right plonker.

'All right, babe?' I asked a purple-faced Vicks with a grin and then dived down the business end with my camera. Everything happened so fast then. I can honestly say that I have never seen so much blood. The surgeon cut the umbilical cord and the nurses held up a screaming 7lb 14oz Dexter so I could take photos. His skin was so red that I told Vicky with a laugh, 'He looks like he's wearing a Man United shirt!'

I was still grinning away when a nurse unexpectedly dumped him in my arms so that she could help to stem Vicky's bleeding.

'Stay with us!' one of the doctors said.

'I'm not going anywhere!' I replied, thinking they were talking to me. Looking up, I realised that there was something seriously wrong and that Vicky had lost consciousness. Holding our wriggling son as he exercised his impressive lungs, I watched the medical team and could tell from the way they were barking orders to each other that this was life-threatening.

'There's no time to cross match her!' someone shouted. 'Get me some universal blood.'

As I stood helplessly to one side, I thought, 'Fucking hell. Vicks might not make it here.' In all our discussions about end-of-life choices and the decisions we needed to make in preparation for my death, we'd never factored in the possibility that she might die first.

It took them several minutes to stabilise her but they finally did, thank goodness. When someone eventually remembered that I was still in the room holding Dex, they took him from me and ushered me outside to wait. It seemed an age before Vicky was moved to a ward where I could see her, and she was very poorly. The doctors had accidentally cut her bladder, for which she needed all sorts of additional procedures later. Then she developed sepsis and cellulitis and was in hospital for quite some time.

Finally, looking very pale, she came home with Dex on 14 February 2015. It was almost exactly one year to the day since we'd met at Andy Harrison's leaving party. So much had been thrown at us in that single year that it was difficult to take everything in – or was that just me? We'd fallen in love, planned my bike ride, found out that Vicks was pregnant, learned that the symptoms of my dementia had begun, been given the bad news by the Army, lost Mum, and very nearly lost Vicky.

Now, back home with Dex, we could breathe a collective sigh of relief and try to put all that behind us at last. That 14 February was, without doubt, the best Valentine's Day ever. Curled up together and so happy to have her home, the two of us stared in wonder at what we'd created in Dexter Anthony Graham.

No matter what his genetic make-up was or what life threw at us next, we had inadvertently given each other the best anniversary and Valentine's gift with our perfect little boy.

If in doubt – take life one day at a time.

15

'If you don't know where you are going
any road will get you there.'
LEWIS CARROLL

Dementia Adventure Diary, 12 December 2015, Brighton, Ontario, Canada

Even though I was more than ready to get back to my little family after eight months on the road, I was still determined to reach Halifax, Nova Scotia and the furthest point north-east on my big journey. It felt like it was the last thing I had to achieve.

I'm sure Vicks and everyone else thought I was bonkers. We had no money, I was emotionally and physically exhausted (as was she), and she was worried that my insistence on heading to the frozen North might delay me getting home for Christmas. To her credit, she didn't complain and continued to encourage me in every way.

After a night with the mother-in-law of a friend in Boston on 26 November, I headed north into New Hampshire and past the superb city of Manchester, named after my own great metropolis and listed as the thirteenth best place to live in the USA. Only thirteenth? Are they sure?

Then I moved on towards Maine, the 'Pine Tree State'. By the end of November my sitrep was a photo of me shivering by a state sign having just arrived, and complaining that it was so cold I couldn't feel my face. I added, 'If in doubt – Freeeeeeeze!'

Vicky commented, 'Suck it up, princess. You have teething, night feeds and stinky nappies to look forward to when you get back to the UK.'

Pushing on towards the maritime province of New Brunswick in freezing rain, I complained that it was very hard going and that Shirley and I were soaked through. Loads of people commented, wishing me luck and telling me to keep dry and stay safe. My sister Lizzie wrote: 'Well done for keeping going. The end is near; the finish line is in sight. Head down and push through it. We're all behind you, pushing you through!'

When I posted a photo of my mum, Lizzie wrote: 'Mum and Dad are with you every step and pedal of the way, Chris. As are we all.' My sister Ange added, 'Mum will be bursting with pride in heaven,' and my half-sister Alison commented: 'Mum will be telling everyone about her amazing son.'

Someone emailed me a cartoon of Santa and Rudolf the reindeer broken down at the side of the road with Rudolf telling someone on the phone: *What can I say? Weather's crap. Sledge is buggered. Fatty's in a strop – just another Christmas really.* It made me laugh so hard that I had to post it online.

The further north and east I went, the colder it became. New Brunswick's provincial motto translates to 'Hope Restored', but my hopes of getting all the way to Nova Scotia were fading fast the closer I got. The freezing rain turned to sticky wet sleet and then proper flakes of snow. Many of the minor roads had already been closed for the winter and I wasn't allowed on the highways, which were down to two tyre tracks in the sub-zero temperatures and four-inch drifts. I had no choice but to load Shirley onto a Greyhound bus to see if we could get through further up another way, but instead I reached a traveller's rest stop at a town called Houlton on the border, where I was gutted to find the weather had closed in still further and there was a foot of the white stuff.

About turn.

'We have a slight problem because – look,' I reported somewhat glumly online on 4 December before panning my camera round. 'I think someone's got dandruff, but as you can see it's snow. I'm not sure what I'm going to do. All I can do is sleep on it and see what the crack is in the morning. The only thing I can do now is make a snowman. Well, it is winter isn't it, eh?'

In spite of my enforced lightheartedness, I was gutted because I knew in my heart that getting the

350 miles to Halifax in 'New Scotland' was no longer feasible. Even more of the roads had been closed due to the snowfall and were impassable for anything but snow ploughs and four-wheel drive vehicles, which meant that they'd be completely out of the question for a bike. Eventually, I had no choice but to admit defeat. I posted online, 'Hello Dementia Adventure friends. Just to inform you, I have about turned. I will not be completing the last little hop to Nova Scotia due to the weather ... clearly cycling in deep snow with narrow bike tyres is not a good or safe thing to do. I am now heading back down the coast towards Toronto. Safety first. It is a slip and slide day.'

The following morning, and with a heavy heart, Shirley and I headed south-west towards the 'Granite State' of New Hampshire. My route would take me on through the 'green mountains' of Vermont, before dipping briefly into Quebec and dropping down to Ontario and my imaginary finishing line back in Brighton.

It seemed impossible to grasp that I only had seven hundred or so miles to go before I rode back down the street where Dean and Nicole Stokes lived. That was a distance I could probably manage in seven days, weather permitting. From the moment I turned away from the New Brunswick border, my cycle back to base camp Stokes felt quite different to anything I had done before. The state motto for Quebec is *Je Me Souviens*, 'I Remember', and it was certainly a time of reflection for me.

I was not only on the home straight but I was heading back to the UK and to my family, and a

254

whole new way of life now that I was officially no longer in the Army. Ten days after my return, on 4 January, I would also be forty years old – a milestone birthday that most people celebrate with a combination of relief at having made it and a sense of trepidation at reaching middle age. My feelings about being in my fifth decade were very different. My dad had died at forty-two, and Tony was dying at forty-three. In 2014, the Army doctors had told me they thought I had seven years left, which meant that by 2016 my allotted timespan would have shrunk to five.

Only five more years of life, if I was lucky and didn't have a fall like my brother or develop the symptoms of a stroke. Natalie and Marcus would be young adults by then, but Dexter would be about the same age at my death as I was when my father died. I have virtually no memories of Dad aside from him drinking from a bottle of Fairy Liquid, so what would Dex remember about me? Not anything like that, I hoped.

One thing I know for sure is that Vicky and my sisters would never allow my memory to fade the way that Mum did with our father. There would be photos and videos, articles and – of course – this book. Hopefully all my kids will read it one day and be proud, or maybe they'll just think, 'Daft bugger!' Even so, I hope that they'll realise that I didn't take my diagnosis lying down and tried to make the most of the time I had left. And that I did all I could in my final years to offer myself to medical science, promote awareness, and raise money for research which might help their future wellbeing.

My journey around North America had undoubtedly become something of an obsession for me and provided a much-needed distraction from the horrors we'd recently faced. From the day Dean left me in Ontario to cycle on alone, I'd been determined to battle on solo against the odds. I'd survived the massive RVs and the giant bull-nose Peterbilt trucks. I'd ridden through plagues of insects that had almost driven me to the brink of insanity. I'd somehow managed not to get eaten by a bear, murdered by a serial killer, struck by lightning, hospitalised with prostatitis, mugged, stampeded by bison, stung by a scorpion, or fried to a crisp in the desert. I hadn't fallen off and broken any bones, been bitten by a rattlesnake, died of dehydration, or been defeated by food poisoning.

Thanks largely to Vicky I had found my way along a complicated 16,000-mile circuit of highways and side roads, back streets and cycle paths. I was treated like a prince by most of the people I'd met and been humbled by their generosity and their own sad stories of dementia. Complete strangers had welcomed me into their homes or vehicles; they'd fed me, donated money to the cause, helped pay for things or supported me from afar. Vicky's parents had been fantastic with the kids when she was knackered and kept us afloat when funds were low, and people like Pete Davies and Craig Calder had stepped in too in remarkable ways. Men and women I didn't even know had completed a run or cycled miles in order to raise money for me and I could never thank them enough because their small acts of kindness meant so much.

I had also been completely overcome by the sheer scale of this planet that I'd longed to explore since I was a kid in geography class at school. I'd surpassed all those boyhood ambitions, camping out under the stars and seeing some unforgettable sights, not least the way the sun resolutely rises and sets regardless of all our hopes and dreams. I was one tiny human being pedalling furiously away across the surface of that vast continent; at one with nature and communing with wildlife in a way I could never have imagined.

Perhaps most tellingly, eight months alone with my mind had allowed me to ponder my thirty-nine years of life, from growing up permanently hungry in Bowdon Vale, losing Dad, living in the various children's homes, then into the military and beyond. It hadn't all been rosy, by any means, but so much of it had been an unforgettable and meaningful adventure. In between delivering mail, dodging bullets, building a shanty house and earning my green lid, I'd fathered three fantastic kids who have made me enormously grateful and immensely proud. If they have inherited nothing else from me, I hope they will have my optimistic nature, dogged determination, insatiable curiosity and appetite for adventure. Through them and with Vicky, I can honestly say that I came to a kind of peace with myself and with whatever lies ahead for us all.

Back in Canada, all that lay immediately ahead – incredibly – was the finishing line. As I crossed back over the Ontario border just south of Montreal, I was struck by how many geese there were – all flying south. Poor Vicks soon heard quite enough about them, as I'd call her up again and again just to cry in wonder, 'I don't believe it, babes. There's even more geese now. Look, there's hundreds of them. The sky looks like the Battle of Britain. Listen to them all!'

Posting a video about it, I said, 'I am now back in Canada, which it is good to be. Although it's a little noisy these days, especially in the morning because there's thousands and thousands of Canadian geese all buggering off to Africa for the summer to get away from the Canadian winter. You can't blame them though, to be fair. It's not a bad life, eh? They get a free flight, they don't have to worry about bombers going to blow the plane up and they get a good seat. Genius move. I might come back as one of them, reincarnated.'

Vicks was far too excited about me almost being home to worry about what I might come back as in the next life. She wrote on my Facebook page: 'Update from Mission Control: Arriving at Finish Line in Brighton Ontario 3 p.m. Local Time (8 p.m. UK time) – Barring no more snow/bike/route disasters Chris is now tracking to cross the finish line Friday 11 December. 187 miles to go!! Track Chris on his final leg.'

Sensing her excitement, I posted a favourite photo of us together in Vancouver and commented: 'Without this woman, Victoria Holmes, I wouldn't be on the last leg of the bike ride. She is my rock and I love her more than she knows xxxx'.

Nobody but me knows just how much she did for me in terms of keeping me company and boosting my spirits, day and night. We hardly even knew each other before she blindly accepted

258

me, my terminal diagnosis, and the fact that – even with the clock ticking – I'd be spending a year of it away from her and our newborn. My madcap adventure must have shaved about a minute off our five minutes of amazing, and yet still she never complained. On the contrary, she carried on supporting and encouraging me to the final second.

When she saw the photo I'd put online, she wrote: 'Awww, I just woke up to this. Now I'm bawling. I love this picture and I love you with all my heart and soul xxx I would not change this journey or you for the whole world. Can't wait for you to come home xxxx'.

I couldn't either, but first there was the small matter of pushing myself for the final few days. From the road south of Montreal, it was downhill and south-west in a chilly wind towards towns like Lancaster and Cornwall, Winchester and Inverary. What with the terrible weather and the place names, it was no wonder I was getting ever more homesick. At T minus one, on what was still 10 December for me, Vicks put up a video in which she couldn't stop grinning from ear to ear. 'Good afternoon Dementia Adventure friends. This is Victoria from Mission Control. I can hardly believe that this is going to be the last time that I'll make a check in or an update or anything like that on the website.

'He's crossing that finish line in about eight hours, which will be seven thirty to eight o'clock UK time and two thirty to three o'clock local time. I'm going to be guiding him in so I'll get to share that moment with him on the phone. I know I speak for hundreds of you who have been following his journey when I say proud doesn't even do it justice. He is phenomenal. I'm not really sure what I'm going to be doing with myself in the evenings now. Maybe something normal like watching television. Looking forward to getting Chris back for our little boy Dexy... The count-down has started but this is not the end... Much love to all of you for your support, we couldn't have done it without you. Merry Christmas.'

In the next few hours, she went on to report 'Sixty minutes', then 'Thirty minutes', before put-ting up a video of Europe singing 'The Final Countdown'. I meanwhile was oblivious to all this, pedalling away, seeing the signs for Brighton and not quite believing them. Needing a pit stop for the last night, I stayed with Dean's mother-in-law Phyllis Da Silva in a town called Brockville, Ontario, 120 miles out of Brighton, where I was fed and fed until I was fit to burst. The next morning, with a full belly after a big breakfast, I was in no particular hurry, so I sauntered into Trenton, nine miles outside Brighton, and stopped at the bike shop that had kindly serviced Shirley when I'd first flown into Canada back in April.

'I'll come and see you on my way home for a cup of tea and tell you all about it,' I'd told the owner Sandy and the mechanic Craig, and they'd promised to hold me to it. They wouldn't have expected me much before April 2016 but, much to their surprise, there I stood in the doorway – eleven stone of fighting muscle, asking for a cup of Rosy Lee. They were very enthusiastic as I told them all about my adventure and I was so glad

I'd stopped by.

Meanwhile, Dean and Vicky were virtually pulling their hair out. Unbeknown to me, Dean had arranged a welcome committee, so people were standing around outside his house waiting for my triumphant return. Vicky and he had conspired to get me there at a certain time with a few strategic stops so that I didn't arrive too soon. My unplanned visit to the bike shop put a literal spanner in the works.

'What are you doing, Chris? Where are you?' Vicky asked me in an urgent call. 'You need to get to Dean's – now!'

I put on my helmet and clipped in my feet and set off at a lazy pace along Main Street, then turned left onto Ontario Street and into the leafy residential area I soon recognised. By the time I prepared to turn into Dean's road I was feeling pretty mellow, although it still hadn't sunk in that my Dementia Adventure was about to come to an end.

Vicky was alongside me, figuratively speaking, as I told her where I was, and how far from Dean and Nicole's house.

'Oh my God, Chris, you've almost made it!' she squealed.

The sight that met me when I did turn the corner almost stopped me mid-pedal. The street was crowded with people waving and smiling and taking photos. There were balloons and streamers, reporters, and a bunch of kids from the local school. Dean had printed some flyers and invited his friends and his running chums. He'd also canvassed his neighbours door to door to tell them all about me and ask them to come out onto the street to welcome me back. Almost everyone did.

I was speechless and emotional all at once as I pedalled Shirley through the purple ribbon strung across the road to signify the final line. Everyone was clapping and cheering and whistling, and Vicky was in tears listening to it all. 'Bloody con-gratulations, babes!' she said, whooping and yelling in my ear.

It was hard to describe the jumbled emotions I felt inside at that moment. I was still buzzing from my experience of a lifetime, but also strangely anxious about what coming to the end of my journey would mean. The appearance of so many strangers caught me by surprise and, for once, I was momentarily lost for words.

Dean and Nicole rushed forward to welcome me with hugs. Ever since I'd first told him of my diagnosis in Sierra Leone in 2010, Dean had been such a great support. 'I thought only old people got dementia?' he'd said, until I explained. My news clearly came as a massive shock to him and he asked bitterly, 'How come only the good die young?' I told him not to worry about it and from then on, we always laughed it off together, joking about what I did and didn't remember – like the tenner he claims to have lent me!

Dean introduced me to the mayor of Brighton, who shook my hand as the cameras rolled. Someone was there from the town newspaper. So, still grinning, I posed for photographs, thumbs up, and with a smiling 'Sausages!' It was all a bit overwhelming for the kid from the Vale.

Still straddling my bike and facing my public

once all the applause had died down, I said, 'I'd like to thank you all for turning out. I really appreciate it. The idea of this bike ride was to raise awareness for dementia research. They say that one in three people on this planet will get some sort of dementia or Alzheimer's, so hopefully I'm getting awareness out there and better treatment for those in old folks' homes around the world because some of them aren't the best and it's a slow death. It's a big problem in society and it costs lots and lots of money for every country in the world ... and it's clogging up everything. Hopefully soon, we'll get a cure. I'm going to carry on doing some charity work and we'll get there. Merry Christmas and have a Happy New Year!'

Dean and Nicole had prepared loads of food and drink for everyone, and there was no shortage of takers. I was so happy that I'd made it back in one piece that I couldn't stop grinning from ear to ear. I even drank a celebratory beer. When the mayor realised that Vicky was online with me, he asked to say a few words. She was a bit nonplussed when he started chatting away to her – because, unbeknown to him, she was breastfeeding Dex at the time.

Dean introduced me to one of his neighbours, Steve, a man in his fifties who has the same kind of early-onset dementia as me, only more advanced. Even though he couldn't walk very well, he and his family came out to welcome me back and we had a brief chat. It was humbling, but bittersweet, because just at the point when I was revelling in the moment, the vacant look in

Steve's eyes once again reminded me of Tony and what lay in my immediate future.

When all the excitement had died down and I'd had a few days to allow my body and mind to rest, the immensity of what I'd achieved in the previous eight months finally sank in. As usual Vicky summed it up well when she posted online: '16,000 miles. Just to put this in perspective, it is just under 18,000 miles to Australia and back, 25,000 miles around the globe via the equator, and just under 12,500 miles North Pole to South Pole. Temperatures ranging from 125° heat to -10° cold. 238 days cycling. 8,000,568 pedal turns. One man, one bike, one mission, well and truly accomplished!'

When she put it like that, I was really chuffed with myself and so proud of Vicks for coming through for me time and again. All that we had been through together would probably have destroyed most relationships, but it had only made ours stronger. I couldn't wait to get home in two weeks' time and thank her in person.

But first, I had some sightseeing to do. Ever since I'd seen the movie *Superman II* when I was six years old and watched Clark Kent launch into superhero mode to heroically rescue a little boy from the thundering waters of Niagara Falls, I'd wanted to visit them for myself. I couldn't have made it on Shirley in the snow, but Dean was happy to drive me the five hundred mile round trip so that I could fulfil a childhood dream. The falls didn't disappoint one little bit. What an astonishing and noisy spectacle they are. Best of all, I could finally buy myself my first small memento of my 16,000-mile journey. Yes, you guessed it – a Niagara Falls fridge magnet. What else?

With that ticked off my list, all I had to do was mark time until my pre-booked flight (that sadly couldn't be altered so close to Christmas) and give my hyped-up metabolism a chance to settle. It was still in overdrive and meant I was still eating for four. After eight months of consuming several times more food than usual, it would take me a while to get used to the notion of only having one plate at a time. Fortunately, Dean and Nicole are feeders, so I just kept devouring all that they put in front of me until I found my way back to some level of normality.

It also took me a week or so to rid myself of the routines of getting up before dawn and planning the next leg of my journey. It even felt strange to walk again, putting one leg in front of the other to achieve forward motion without two wheels spinning beneath me. With nothing to fill my time, all I could do was wash my sweat-stained Lycra, pack my case, and get ready to fly home for Christmas.

By the Left!

A big family reunion was lined up, as well as multi-media appearances, including a turn on BBC *Breakfast,* and – just in time – I heard the fantastic news from Alzheimer's Research that I had not only reached my £40,000 target but topped it by more than £11,000, with more still coming in. I'd raised at least £51,000! I could hardly believe it.

'What will you do next?' everyone began to ask

me, and it was a question I was already asking myself as I started to feel a bit flat after so long on the road. The sense of anti-climax was only compounded by the wait to get home.

'Something closer to home, and only if I can get sponsored this time,' I mused. 'Maybe a run from Land's End to John O'Groats?' That somehow felt too tame after my Dementia Adventure, though, and I wondered what else I might do to raise money for Alzheimer's Research.

Nothing fazed Vicky much, and she didn't even flinch when I started talking about my next fundraiser. As she always said, we're two peas in a pod in terms of our love of excitement and have been through so much in such a short time that we find it a bit unsettling when things go back to 'normal'. Besides, she was always one hundred per cent behind anything I chose to do with the last few years of my life.

The only time I heard her gasp in shock and horror was when I said, almost in passing, during one of our daily Skype chats from Canada, 'Maybe I could cycle around the world's biggest island?'

'What? Where, Chris? You don't mean – Australia?' Her eyes virtually came out on stalks.

'Uh-huh. That would be something, wouldn't it?'

'Over my dead body, soldier!' she cried. 'And probably yours. I'm not being your satnav for that! What are you thinking?'

'Well, at least I can cycle now, and I could probably master a map or two on my own. So job done, right?'

'No!' she said, putting her foot down. 'And

anyway, it's too far. You need to think of something much closer to home.'

It didn't take long for her to come up with a plan. Within days, she came back to me with, 'Guess what, Chris? There are two hundred and sixty-seven inhabited islands around Great Britain...'

'There are?'

'Yes. And you love kayaking.'

She was right. I'd done a bit in some rivers in Wales during an adventure-training course, as well as on Ascension Island in the South Atlantic while I was based in the Falklands. I'd mastered forward motion and could probably survive a roll or two. What else did I need to know?

'At least if you were kayaking around the UK then we could all come and see you and even do a bit with you,' she reasoned.

'That would be great!' I cried, as the light bulb finally switched on in my brain.

If in doubt – paddle?

Epilogue

'Lean forward to the next crazy adventure beneath the skies.'

JACK KEROUAC

Dementia Adventure Diary, summer 2016, Mission Control, Brize Norton, England

There had been no fuss or fanfare the day I'd left the Army. I'd received my citation for 'exemplary service', turned down the chance to be dined out in the sergeants' mess, gifted my dress uniform to a charity shop and simply walked away from the life I'd loved.

Dismissed!

My feelings of sorrow and disappointment weren't much helped by the fact that the RAF doctor who conducted my last medical before I hung up my boots told me she thought I was in excellent shape and that if I'd been in the Air Force, they'd have kept me on in some capacity or other until the bitter end.

By the time the military had worked out my medical pension and all the monies I was due, I received a final lump sum of £38,000 (a huge chunk of which had been spent funding my bike ride). If I hadn't admitted to my condition and carried on in service until the end after my promotion to warrant officer second class, that amount would have been closer to £60,000. I had to be happy with what I was given and the eight campaign medals I had to show for my years in the armed forces, including for Bosnia, Kosovo, Afghanistan, and working for Air Corps Iraq, plus a commander's commendation or two.

I may not be the sharpest tool in the box but I should have suspected that my loyal shipmates wouldn't be happy with such an unsatisfactory ending for my military career. It was Pete Davies who told Vicks how gutted he and the lads were that I didn't have a dine out. She had already hatched a plan to throw me a surprise homecoming and fortieth, as I'd never had a big birthday party in my life. As I'd explained to her, being born at the beginning of January was crap timing because everyone was always too exhausted and skint from Christmas and the New Year to help me celebrate.

Vicky wasn't going to let me get away without a party though, so when she cheekily asked Pete if it could be held in the sergeants' mess in South Cerney, he rallied the troops and the two of them set me up good and proper. Inviting me to the mess for 'a drink with a few of the lads' on 9 January 2016, five days after my fortieth birthday, Pete and Vicks arranged for a hundred and thirty people from all phases of my life to be waiting. Pete even created a short video, featuring photos of my ride and career, which he posted on YouTube to advertise the party. It was titled *Chris Graham – The Legend Returns*.

A few paces in front of Vicks, I walked un-suspectingly into the mess that night (I was late, of course) and couldn't believe the huge crowd forming a vanguard of applause, camera flashes and cheers. Gobsmacked and more than a little overwhelmed, I did a forward victory roll on the carpet just to break the ice.

It was such a fantastic party with so many friends and family, including my sisters and their families, who had travelled all the way from Manchester. Tony's ex-wife Jan came from Wales, and my schoolfriend Rachel Curwen was there too, along with so many other old faces that I genuinely struggled to remember them all. There was a subsidised bar, a disco and a charity raffle. The walls were plastered with photos of my bike ride, of my early days in the Army and of me growing up, and Pete arranged for an official photographer to take loads of memorable shots.

Major Ian Booth, the man who'd known me all my military career and persuaded 'Desperate Dan' to let me try for my green beret many years earlier, gave a very amusing speech, beginning with, 'I promise to keep this as short as Chris and Vicky's sex life ... so goodnight everyone!'

His promised character assassination of 'our little Gurkha postie' ended up being far from it. I was quite choked by the end. Boothy said, 'We are here to celebrate Chris's remarkable achievement and his safe return from his cycling adventure and, of course, to ensure he actually leaves the Army with the send-off he so rightly deserves.'

He added that the last time he'd seen so many posties was in a court martial. Of me he said, 'I have watched him mature a bit like a cheese – slowly, left in the dark – get promoted, get bust, get promoted, get punched – several times – and finally seen him become a superb soldier and proud father.'

He called me 'determined' and 'resilient', said I thought I was invincible, and spent most of my career 'not working but hiking and climbing around his native Nepal – sorry, I meant Manchester.' He told tales of drunken nights out in foreign parts, including the night he and I got into a punch-up with some nightclub bouncers in Norway. We ended up being arrested by the Norwegian police, who I tried to persuade to release us by saying, 'You can't nick me! I'm from Manchester!' (Astonishingly, that didn't work.)

Major Booth added: 'Chris has enjoyed a remarkable career and the reason we stand here today is to acknowledge a man that is dear to our hearts – you cannot NOT like Chris.'

After I quipped that I couldn't remember a single person in the room, he went on: 'Victoria, you have partnered a man who will offer you total love, devotion and protection. He has and will no doubt continue to drive you to distraction – as he did with most people in this room – but I know everyone will agree that there is no better man you would want as the father of your child or by your side when things get tough. Just don't ask him to add up – it's not his strong point.

Everyone laughed at that, as they did at most of the things Boothy said, but I have to admit to feeling quite emotional when he concluded with, 'Chris, can I just say how proud we all are to have you as a friend and colleague and to witness what has been a truly inspirational bike ride to help others... You are called the Gurkha not only because you look like one but more importantly because you are loyal, dedicated, extremely courageous and proud.' He ended cheekily with, 'I just want to publicly announce that Chris is buying everyone a drink because he is such a generous person! To Chris Graham – legend!'

I gave my response standing on the arms of a chair so that everyone could see me, even at the back of the room. 'I've got dementia,' I said, choking up. 'It's in my family. Shit happens. I thought I could either sit down and mope or get on a bike and cycle. I wanted to raise funds and keep myself fit. I'm a soldier, first and foremost. People think they can't do something but if you break it down, day by day, you can eventually build up and do it. I urge you to keep fit for your health and to do something to raise money for charity.'

As I told everyone that night, it was my avowed intention to look into what I could next do to both fundraise and continue to keep myself in peak condition. I was still fully functioning and bucking the family trend. Although my short-term memory wasn't nearly as good as my long-term memory, my mental decline was much slower than my brother Tony's had been at the same age. The doctors couldn't really explain why that was, but I put it down to my high level of personal fitness. I went for a long run every day and did all I could to eat healthily and live well, including drinking alcohol only very rarely and taking all the recommended supplements Vicky fed me like Smarties to enhance the pro-

272

duction of good chemicals in my brain.

By my age, my father was nearing death and Tony was in hospital, so as long as I could continue to train and keep a healthy supply of blood and oxygen to my brain, I hoped I'd stay sound. Up until I finished my bike ride, I'd never taken any medication for my condition at all, but not long after I returned I went to see Professor Fox, who prescribed me a drug called Donepezil, better known as Aricept, commonly used in the palliative care of people with Alzheimer's. It's not a cure, nor does it slow the progression, but it is supposed to improve cognitive function. The side effects are nausea and stomach upset and – somewhat alarmingly in my case – vivid dreams that have caused me to act out in my sleep occasionally, freaking Vicky out. Nothing new there then.

Vicks thought I was more clear-headed in the mornings since I'd been taking it, but I didn't notice any dramatic changes. I tried taking a higher dose but my body couldn't tolerate it and my head buzzed as if it was radioactive. I felt like a zombie, so I stuck to the lower dosage of 5 mg daily. As time goes on, I hope to be offered some of the new trial therapies that might at least keep me stable.

All I could do in the meantime was think about what I might realistically do next – when not trying to raise money, that is. Shirley was dismantled and packed away in the shed, and I resisted the temptation to go out and chat away to her as I had throughout the previous year. I probably should have sold her as soon as I got home to raise a bit of extra cash, but I couldn't do that quite yet, not

273

after all we'd been through together.

In March 2016, I was made a Champion of Alzheimer's Research UK by the charity for being what they called an 'inspirational cyclist, dedicated fundraiser and spokesperson', someone who'd raised the profile of dementia research. The charity announced, 'The forty-year-old from Oxfordshire completed the challenge ... equipped with nothing more than a bike, a tent and the essential supplies, experiencing extreme temperatures from sub-zero through to a blistering 125 degrees Fahrenheit. However this failed to stop him shaving four months off the trip – completing it in just eight months rather than a year as he had originally anticipated.

'This accolade recognises Chris's exceptional support and bravery in facing dementia head on... We cannot thank him enough.'

I joined a small group of thirty-five fellow champions who have made 'outstanding efforts' to raise money and help Alzheimer's Research in its mission to beat dementia. Hilary Evans, the charity's chief executive, described my adventure as staggering.

My response was unequivocal. 'Even though I know what will happen to me in the coming years, I now have direction in life. I wanted to do something to fight back – to do as much as I can while I can. It's simple for me, you have to hit the enemy directly, so I took on the 16,000-mile cycle to support Alzheimer's Research.'

Being a champion was fantastic, as was being nominated for a Soldiering On award a few weeks later (an honour given to those in the armed forces community), but neither would do much to help me get a paying job. My hopes of joining the civilian post office were no longer practical, given my memory lapses. Although I was still driving, I knew I might not always be able to do so. One thing I did know was that I intended to make an honest woman out of Vicky one day, although I still had to figure out when that might be.

Not long after I returned from Canada, we were discussing our future and I suddenly told her in a very matter-of-fact way, 'We're getting married.'

'Oh, we are, are we?' she replied, laughing.

A couple of weeks later, a news item popped up on my social network feed about Kylie Minogue announcing her recent engagement and flashing a dazzling diamond ring. Thinking that I hadn't heard anything about Kylie in a while, I innocently showed it to Vicky.

'Gorgeous ring,' she commented, somewhat ruefully.

Looking up, I gasped. 'Oh fuck, babes! I forgot to propose, didn't I?'

She nodded and gave me the smile that told me I was forgiven. 'Don't worry, Chris,' she said graciously, 'You've had a lot on your mind lately.'

'But I didn't propose and I can't even afford to buy you a nice ring. I'm such a dick. You can slap me if you like.'

'No need,' she said sweetly. Referring to her beloved grandmother, who'd passed away twenty years ago, she added, 'Mum has kept Nana's engagement ring for me. We can use that.'

'No!' I insisted, jumping up. 'I'm going to buy you your own ring – a proper one. It might not be soon and it won't be like Kylie's, but it will be yours and it'll be from me. Something to have for always.'

'All right,' she said. 'But there's no hurry.'

A few weeks later, I picked my moment. It might not have been quite as romantic as she'd hoped, but I couldn't wait a day longer. It was one in the morning and Vicks was sitting on the living room floor in her pyjamas trying to sort out the nightmare that is my admin backlog after eight months away. When she finally finished she sat back from the pile of paperwork and announced triumphantly, 'Done!'

'What are you doing for the next few years?' I asked with a grin.

Thinking I was referring to her having more time after the madness of the bike ride and trying to sort out the mess of my life, she laughed, until I pulled out her grandmother's diamond and ruby engagement ring and presented it to her with the words, 'How about being my wife?'

Shaking her head at my crap timing, while laughing and crying at the same time, she threw her arms around me and accepted immediately. 'Of course I will, you muppet! Who else would have you?'

We didn't immediately set a date for our wedding because we knew it would be sensible to first figure out what we were going to live on. Vicks is doing her photography and a couple of jobs as well as looking after Dex, Katy and me, and I hope to find something meaningful to do while seeking sponsorship for my next adventure, whatever that might be.

We did settle on a couple of things in this puzzle of a life, though, the first of which was my vasectomy. 'I'm prepared to put my balls on the line for you,' I told Vicks jokingly, but we both knew how deadly important it was that I had the snip. Summoning up my courage, I went for the op in April, watching the whole thing while on local anaesthetic in between telling the surgeon, 'I hope you have a steady hand!'

When I got home from hospital I milked it good and proper, lying in bed while Vicky waited on me hand and foot. 'This is good wife training for you,' I quipped, but she didn't seem to find that very funny. Or I'd call out, 'What letter comes after S in the alphabet, Vicks?'

'T,' she'd reply, while busy changing Dexter's nappy, washing up, or making lunch.

'Oooh, yes please. Milk and two sugars for me!'

Amazingly, she still wanted to marry me and although we didn't know when, we did decide that our reception would be a party for two with champagne at sunrise somewhere with history. And in an ideal world, that date we'd choose would be Friday the 13th.

It was Vicks's mum Lynn who first gave us the idea. She'd often tell us, 'If it wasn't for bad luck then you two wouldn't have any luck at all!'

Her words rang so true that, with delicious irony, we couldn't think of a luckier date to get married than the one which – according to superstition – is the unluckiest day of the year. I mean, what could possibly go wrong? Besides, with Vicky at my side I feel like the luckiest man alive.

To once again quote the wisdom of Andy

Dufresne from *The Shawshank Redemption,* life comes down to a simple choice – 'Get busy living or get busy dying.'

If in doubt?

Trust me, there is no time for doubt.

Just live.

Acknowledgements

There are so many people to thank for helping me with my bike ride, as well as with my life in general. First and foremost, I have to thank Victoria Holmes for everything she has done for me since the day we fell in love. I could never have completed my Dementia Adventure without her support and encouragement and I only hope that I continue to live up to her high hopes for five minutes of amazing.

To my sisters Angie Maddocks and Lizzie Fox I owe a lifelong debt of gratitude for being so supportive and forgiving of my mischievous ways. Thanks also to their partners Colin and Kev and to my half-sister Alison Morris, and to Jan Graham and Jayne Cheetham for taking such good care of my brother Tony. A big shout out to my lovely nephews Richard and James too.

Dean and Nicole Stokes were fantastic hosts at the start and end of my ride and I will always be grateful for their generous hospitality. Craig and Ofelia Calder went above and beyond and I really appreciate their help. Pete Davies was a diamond geezer for flying out to join me for part of my journey and raising money along the way, and I hope I never forget what he did for me. Neil Deadman and Rachel Curwen have been friends since school and were massively helpful and encouraging every step of the way. Vicky's parents Lynn and Ken have been amazing, and her daughter Katy has put up with a great deal since the Gurkha moved into her life.

To the long list of those who have gone out of their way to offer me moral, financial, emotional and physical support over the years, and especially since my diagnosis, I salute you. In no particular order, they include Jason Marshall and Carl Cox, Major Ian Booth, Jason Garrett, Andy Harrison and Jenny, Martin Guiney, Frank and Pascale Henvey, Stan Hogg, Johanne Lacoix, Neil Frain, Den Sng, Jamie Clarke and family, Kev Pellington, the staff at the British Embassy Washington, Mark and Alicia Precious, Doug and Jenny Mason, Phyllis Da Silva, Mandy and Anthony Childs, Ian Malcolm Wallace, Jackie and Les McCullough, Derek Munroe, Ian Moore, Jackie Wilson, BFPS BATUS Canada, WRVS BATUS Canada, Peter Turco, Christine Mueller-Wagner, Claude Richer and son, John Wright, Chelsea and Kevin Cleveland, Ashley and Kevin Bradberry, Jean Thigpin, Kelly Scanlon, John Wright, Emmett Kelly, Lorraine Fischer, Jonathan Grey, the staff at Headley Court, Francis Fox, Mark Black, Craig Bibey, Mountain Mania in Carterton, Tri&Run in Trenton (Canada), Mark Swift, Scott and Viv Lister, Adam Dolan, Mark Bragg, Colin Till and all at ABF The Soldiers' Charity, Paul Rui Penu, Val Goulding, Joan Hill, the BBC, BFBS Forces News, Doc McKee and Iceland Air.

Special thanks to Professor Nick Fox, Dr Phil Weston and the team at the Dementia Research

Centre, London, counsellor Alison Clarke and the medical staff in Manchester, and to Alzheimer's Research UK. Also to all those who competed in the Cotswolds 24 Hour Race on my behalf and to the Witney Rotary Club for cycling the Ridgeway, especially Rosie and Richard Howe.

This book would never have been possible without the warm guidance of literary agent Rory Scarfe of Furniss Lawton, or the enthusiasm of Adam Strange and the team at Little, Brown. Writer Wendy Holden showed Gurkha-style stamina and patience while working with me. How she managed to get this much information out of my brain I'll never know.

I am bound to have forgotten people, but all I can say is that it wasn't intentional. Besides, I have a licence to be confused!

If in doubt – apologise.

Glossary

Bergen – Military rucksack
busies – police (Mancunian expression)
Blighty – Great Britain (Army slang)
blue nose – Manchester City supporter (Manc)
brew – cup of tea (slang)
butty – thick cut sandwich (slang)
callsign – lowly soldier (Army expression)
chin-strapped – exhausted (Army slang)
civvy – civilian (slang)
comms – communications (Army slang)
cream crackered – tired (rhyming slang for knackered)
cut my own detail – make my own way (Army expression)
dead – very (Manc)
footie – football (slang)
fullscrew – full corporal (Army slang)
ginnel – alleyway (Manc)
Just do one, will yer? – Get lost (Manc)
kecks – trousers (slang)
kip – sleep (slang)
Manclish – Manchester English (Manc)
mither – bother (Manc)
muckers – mates (slang)
pavement pizza – vomit (slang)
recce – reconnaissance (informal)

Red – a supporter of Manchester United (Manc)
Rosy Lee – tea (Cockney rhyming slang)
scoff – food (Army slang)
Scooby-Doo – clue (Cockney rhyming slang)
scoops – pints (slang)
scran – food (Manc)
sherbets – drinks (informal)
SitRep – Situation Report (informal)
squaddie – soldier (informal)
square bash – march (Army slang)
sticky fingers – thief (slang)
tea leaf – thief (Cockney rhyming slang)
wet – cup of tea or pint of beer
windbagging – chatting (slang)
yomp – march or pace (Army slang)
zeds – sleep or zzz's (slang)
Zulu – Greenwich Mean Time (Army code)

Lyric Credits

'Tears and Rain': James Blunt, EMI Music Publishing, 2003. By James Blount and Guy Chambers.

'Something I Need': Ben Haenow, Kobalt Music Publishing LTD., Universal Music Publishing Group, 2014. By Ryan Tedder and Benjamin Levin.

'You're the Voice': John Farnham, Warner/Chappell Music INC., 1986. By Andy Quanta, Keith Reid, Maggie Ryder and Chris Thompson.

'Happy': Pharrell Williams, PeerMusic Publishing, Sony/ATV Music Publishing LLC, 2013. By Pharrell Williams.

'I Will Follow You Into the Dark': Deathcab for Cutie, Warner/Chappell Music INC., 2006. By Benjamin Gibbard.

'We Found Love': Rihanna, Universal Music Publishing Group, 2011. By Calvin Harris.

'Price Tag': Jesse J, Universal Music Publishing

Group, 2011. By Jessica Cornish,
Lukasz Gottwald, Claude Kelly,
Bobby Ray Simmons, Jr.

'Iris': Goo Goo Dolls, Warner/Chappell Music
INC., 1998. By John Rzeznik.

The publishers hope that this book has given you enjoyable reading. Large Print Books are especially designed to be as easy to see and hold as possible. If you wish a complete list of our books please ask at your local library or write directly to:

Magna Large Print Books
Magna House, Long Preston,
Skipton, North Yorkshire.
BD23 4ND

This Large Print Book for the partially sighted, who cannot read normal print, is published under the auspices of

THE ULVERSCROFT FOUNDATION

THE ULVERSCROFT FOUNDATION

... we hope that you have enjoyed this Large Print Book. Please think for a moment about those people who have worse eyesight problems than you ... and are unable to even read or enjoy Large Print, without great difficulty.

You can help them by sending a donation, large or small to:

**The Ulverscroft Foundation,
1, The Green, Bradgate Road,
Anstey, Leicestershire, LE7 7FU,
England.**
or request a copy of our brochure for more details.

The Foundation will use all your help to assist those people who are handicapped by various sight problems and need special attention.

Thank you very much for your help.